Contents

Acknowledgements

I would like to express my gratitude to all of my fellow Alexander teachers and particularly to Krii Ackers, Mike Birley, Don and Carmen Burton, Jean Clark, Margaret Farrar, Mary Holland, John Nicholls, Frank Sheldon, Jean Shepherd, Robin Simmons, Chris Stevens and Sue Thame.

In addition, I wish to express my special thanks to: Paul Collins and Elizabeth Rajna Collins for creating the opportunity for me to become a teacher of the Alexander Technique and for pioneering the 'Application Approach'; Walter Carrington and Peggy Williams for providing me with a standard of excellence in teaching; Isobel McGilvray for sharing her magic with me; Tony Buzan for his inspiration and vision; and Bridget Belgrave for her love, support and picture research.

I would like to thank the people who contributed to the creation of this book: Diane Aubrey, Angela Caine, Michael Haggiag, Brian Helweg-Larsen, Leah Landau, Ray Martin, Tony Pearce, Christopher Pick, Peter Russell and Mrs Peter Scott.

Preface to the new edition

In the Preface to the new edition of *Man's Supreme Inheritance*, published in 1945, Alexander suggested that many of humanity's problems were attributable to our inability to deal with 'a quickly changing environment'. As we approach the twenty-first century the pace of change has accelerated enormously. Yet Alexander's prescription for meeting the challenges of change has become more relevant than ever. He wrote in the same Preface: 'It is what man *does* that brings the wrong thing about, first within himself and then in his activities in the outside world, and it is only by preventing this doing that he can ever begin to make any real change. In other words, before man can make the changes necessary in the outside world, he must learn to know the kind of doing he should prevent in himself, and the HOW of preventing it. Change must begin in his own behaviour.'

Alexander's emphasis on individual responsibility and prevention is the point of departure for understanding and applying his work. *Body Learning* is intended as inspiration and guidance for those who consider commencing this journey, and as refreshment for those who have been travelling it for a while.

Since *Body Learning* was first published in 1981, readers have asked many questions about the Alexander work. Some are relatively simple: 'How many lessons will I need?' or 'What is the difference betwen the Alexander Technique and the Feldenkrais method?' Others are more complex: 'How does the Alexander Technique affect the emotions?' or 'Can the Alexander Technique improve my interpersonal relationships?' In this new edition I've included my replies to these and many other most commonly asked or interesting questions.

In the first edition I reported on my experience of applying the Alexander Technique to activities ranging from learning to juggle and riding a unicycle, to singing and writing. This new version includes descriptions of applying the Technique to learning to swim, learning the martial art of aikido and building my career as a speaker, seminar leader and organizational consultant. I've also included an Appendix which offers some thoughts on the application of the Alexander work in facilitating organizational change. This new edition also includes instructions on how to practice a very useful procedure for freeing yourself from unnecessary tension. It is called the 'balanced resting state procedure' and I hope you find it helpful.

The original idea of *Body Learning* was to provide readers with a 'whole-brained' introduction to the Alexander Technique: carefully chosen words to stimulate your left-brain and inspiring photographs to nourish your right-brain. Thanks once again to the brilliant photo-research of Bridget Belgrave and the efforts of Aurum Press, the right-brain effort has been given even more complete expression. We have taken the best photographs from the first two editions and combined them with some new offerings. Thanks to: Frank Ottiwell, Riki Alexander, Gabrielle Czaja and Michael Frederick for feedback on the new material; to Beret Arcaya for wonderful lesson exchanges; to Jim MacKenzie for his fine photography; to Nusa Maal Gelb for love and support. Special thanks to Sheila Murphy for her help in creating this new edition.

Foreword to the second edition

'Cast away opinion: thou are saved.' Marcus Aurelius is not alone in advising us to let go, to be free, fresh, new – to be *present*. But opinions are not only an intellectual, conscious decision. Opinions are often based on the earliest unconscious conditioning involving our real or imagined safety and even survival. Opinions are deeply entangled in our muscles, in our bones, in our cells. How can such a deep change as 'casting away opinions' take place? How do we differentiate between opinions that are necessary and those that are inappropriate?

Techniques for self-improvement and liberation have been with us for centuries, in the last thirty years a bounty of them has flowered. This abundance presents us with the puzzling choice between being their victims or their beneficiaries.

The Alexander Technique reaches the heart of the question and it does so most subtly: a few words, no calisthenics, no dogma. In this book, each facet of the Work is presented in clear and easy form – a particularly difficult task when describing non-verbal experience. The illustrations are magnificent and illuminating.

Going to church on Sunday is not the essence of religion. Similarly, there is no specific activity which is the essence of the Alexander Technique, for it applies to all living. In the outstanding chapter 'Learning How to Learn', Gelb shows how the Alexander principle is applicable to juggling, speedreading, singing, running and other totally diverse activities.

The Alexander Technique is not a method to accumulate information nor the art of learning something new. It is, instead, the art of *unlearning,* which is much more subtle and, sometimes, a more difficult endeavour – unlearning that which is habitual, instead of natural; letting go of old patterns and of those repetitious opinions arrived at in times and circumstances totally different from those of the present.

Aldous Huxley, my late husband, was enamoured of knowledge – but he was also a master in the art of unlearning.

Maria, Aldous's first wife, wrote to their publisher who had asked if Aldous knew Alexander:

> ... not only does Aldous know about Alexander but goes to him each day since Autumn. He believes he has made a very important, in fact, essential discovery. He certainly has made a new and unrecognizable person of Aldous, not physically only, but mentally and therefore morally. Or rather, he has brought out, actively, all we, Aldous' best friends, know never came out either in the novels or with strangers.

In 1950, Aldous wrote to the French writer Dr Hubert Benoit:

> ... still better were those techniques developed in England by F.M. Alexander, whose books are well worth reading. Alexander discovered empirically, in experimentation on himself, that there is a correct or 'natural' relationship between the neck and the trunk and that normal functioning of the total organism cannot take place except when the neck and the trunk are in this right relationship. His findings have been confirmed theoretically by various physiologists and, in practice, in the persons of the numerous pupils he has taught during the last forty-five years. (I myself am one of his pupils.) For some obscure reason the great majority of those who have come in contact with urbanized, industrial civilization tend to lose the innate capacity for preserving the correct relation between the neck and trunk, and consequently never enjoy completely normal organic functioning. Alexander and the teachers he has trained re-establish the correct relationship and teach their pupils to preserve it consciously. This, as I know by experience, is an exceedingly valuable technique ... practising this awareness makes it possible for the physical organism to function as it ought to function, thus improving the general state of physical and mental health.

For myself, being made aware of the Alexander work and applying it (when I do!) is one of the great gifts Aldous gave me.

LAURA HUXLEY
Los Angeles, California

Foreword
to the first
edition

A famous American author was once asked whether he had ever read any of F. Matthias Alexander's books. He replied, 'No, I don't read books.' And then he paused and gave a slow smile and added: 'You see, I'm a juggler with words myself.'

Michael Gelb is a juggler too; and not only with words. How he came to be so, and to ride a unicycle, and to master a number of other practical skills, is part of the fascinating story told in this book.

An ever-increasing number of people have heard of the Alexander Technique and have even had some practical experience of it, and thus there is a growing demand for more information. Michael Gelb supplies this very well. He does not claim to have written a definitive work, but he offers a clear, contemporary introduction, based on his own experience of applying the Technique in everyday life.

To write about practical procedures is always unsatisfactory and can even be misleading, in as much as the written word cannot convey the relevant experiences: that is why practical skills cannot be properly learned from books alone. Books can inform, stimulate and entertain, but they cannot instruct unless the writer and the reader share at least some amount of experience in common. For the proper understanding and evaluation of practical experience, however, supplementary information is usually necessary. We need to know 'why?' as well as 'how?'. The practice of the Alexander Technique introduces people to many new and unfamiliar experiences, and in order to grasp their implications people need to have as much information as possible.

When you are confronted by the problem of how to do anything, how to juggle for instance, you soon realize that it is a mind–body problem and that you really know very little of the processes involved. The mind obviously affects the body, but the body equally affects the mind. You soon begin to understand that what you *think* is as important as what you *do*. You have to control thinking as well as doing. But since the mind and body together make up the self, the problem can literally be described as a problem of self-control. How is this achieved? The daily process of living goes on for each of us, and, so far as we are aware of what is happening, we say 'yes' to it, or 'no', giving or withholding consent. To some degree at least we do have a conscious choice. Yet when we come to the problem of doing something, as we understand 'doing', how do we make our choice? How do we use ourselves to do it? This was the crucial problem that Alexander posed when he made his classic self-observations: and his answer was that we do not know, any more than the dog or the cat knows.

But we need to know; because the way we use ourselves determines the way in which the whole of our mind–body functions. Mostly we use ourselves in accordance with our habits; we do what has become habitual, and we do and think in the habitual way. As life flows on we react to situations and demands entirely predictably. We give consent to what is going on without any conscious realization of what we are doing. However, our habits often produce all sorts of harmful consequences: stress, strain, nervous tension and ill health. Above all they frequently result in poor posture and movement, poor breathing and digestion. We lose poise, and this tends to handicap us mentally as well as physically. When we encounter the unfamiliar and unknown, we are thrown out of our way, we are at a loss, and we do not know how to react. We strive to make efforts, but mostly they are misdirected and therefore quite counterproductive. This was Alexander's own experience: this was the problem that he recognized. Poise is a fundamental human need. We must have control, conscious, reasoned control of our reactions, but primarily we must learn to control the mechanism of poise; and this necessitates both practical experience and knowledge. It also requires a technique, and this was what Alexander evolved from his self-experiments.

Michael Gelb illuminates the problem from his own experience and observation and makes the implications easier to grasp.

We are all too familiar with the stiffness, tension and futile effort that so often go first into the attempted mastery of a new skill. (Let anyone remind themselves by trying to juggle three balls into the air.) To find a better way must be welcome, and yet surely the most serious concern for human beings today is not so much our limited practical skill or frequent failure to achieve our desired aims as our general state of poor health and the harm and damage that we manifestly suffer in ourselves as we go through life. Our bad habits of mind and body become more entrenched and we feel incapable of doing anything about them. We come to accept this state of affairs as inevitable with a mixture of self-pity and fatalism. Alexander used to say that self-pity needs to give way to self-accusation. We have the power to choose what we do: at least, we have the power to choose what we will *not* do.

If this is so, and we are able to choose how to use ourselves, we cannot afford to let this choice go by default. We must find out how to make change; we must become aware of how we use ourselves and furthermore discover how we *ought* to use ourselves. Otherwise we shall live out our lives as mere slaves of habit and pawns of chance. The Alexander Technique, which this book is about, offers a different prospect: it proposes a means whereby the necessary changes can be made.

WALTER CARRINGTON
Director of The Constructive Teaching Centre, London

Introduction

'What is the Alexander Technique and how can it help me?' I have heard this question hundreds of times since I myself first asked it in 1972. I discovered that it was easy to find out what the Technique was *not*. According to friends who had studied Alexander's work, it was not like yoga, massage or Eastern psychophilosophy; it did not involve doing exercises, and it was much more sophisticated than posture or relaxation training. My friends suggested that I would never really understand what the Technique was about until I took some lessons. I did, and then I began to appreciate their difficulty in defining and describing it.

The Alexander Technique eludes precise definition because it involves a new experience – the experience of gradually freeing oneself from the domination of fixed habits. Any attempt to put that experience into words is necessarily limited, rather like trying to explain music to someone who has never heard a note. Nevertheless I thought the attempt worth making, if only because previous descriptions of the Technique seemed more restricted than necessary and I sensed that it might be possible to stretch the limits of the printed word. The book I have written is the book I wanted when I started to study the Technique.

This book started life as a thesis presented as part of my Master's degree, when I was also in the middle of training as an Alexander teacher. The thesis was written in a somewhat tentative style and was full of phrases such as 'I think' and 'it can be said that'. Since presenting my thesis, I have qualified as an Alexander teacher and have gained a great deal of experience in the Technique. My understanding of it has deepened and its practice has become an integral part of my daily life. In rewriting the manuscript for publication, I have added some descriptions of my experiences as a teacher and have taken great pleasure in removing those tentative phrases, for where once I wrote 'I think', I now find I know. So, what is the Alexander Technique?

The best formal definition is that offered by Dr Frank Jones, former director of the Tufts University Institute for Psychological Research. He described the Technique as 'a means for changing stereotyped response patterns by the inhibition of certain postural sets'.[1] He also described it as 'a method for expanding consciousness to take in inhibition as well as excitation (i.e. "not doing" as well as "doing") and thus obtaining a better integration of the reflex and voluntary elements in a response pattern'.[2] But my favourite definition is the one coined by Gertrude Stein's brother Leo, who called the Technique 'the method for keeping your eye on the ball applied to life'.[3]

The Alexander Technique can help people in several different ways. Much depends on what they need and what they hope to achieve. In general, people seem to take Alexander lessons for three main reasons.

First, pain: people with bad backs, stiff necks, asthma, headaches, depression and many other ailments often find their way to an Alexander teacher's door having exhausted more conventional methods of treatment. These ailments are frequently the result of bad habits of movement and can be relieved through re-education.

Second, performance arts and skill development: bad habits, often the result of general patterns of misuse in daily life, can become exaggerated when one regularly practises a difficult or delicate activity. Breathless actors, violinists with paralysed left shoulders, dancers with back pain and sportsmen with tennis elbow are all suffering from the stress and tension characteristics of their activities and benefit from studying the Technique. Those seeking to master such pursuits can learn by observing the truly great performers, who often display a sense of ease and economy of movement that seems entirely natural. When Artur Rubinstein plays the piano, when Fred Astaire dances, or when Michael Jordan plays basketball, they all have one thing in common: they make it look easy. Alexander discovered that this quality of relaxation in action is not only the result of natural talent but can also be learned.

Third, personal transformation: the development in recent years of humantistic psychology and the increasing popularity of Eastern philosophies have brought about a growing understanding of the importance of the individual's responsibility for the development of his own awareness. In this connection, John Dewey, the American educational philosopher and one of Alexander's most influential supporters, has written:

> The hardest thing to attend to is that which is closest to ourselves, that which is most constant and familiar. And this closest something is, precisely, ourselves, our own habits and ways of doing things.... Never before, I think, has there been such an acute consciousness of the failure of all remedies and forces external to the individual man. It is, however, one thing to teach the need of a return to the individual man as the ultimate agency in whatever mankind and society can collectively accomplish.... It is another thing to discover the concrete procedure by which this greatest of all tasks can be executed. And this indispensable thing is exactly what Mr Alexander has accomplished.[4]

It is almost one hundred years since Alexander first presented his unique insights into the role of the body in the development of conscious learning, yet many people are just now finding that Alexander's work is a powerful tool for heightening self-knowledge and changing habit. In addition, they are also discovering that it is an invaluable tool in the pursuit of such disciplines as yoga, meditation and the martial arts.

Of course, in reality, the distinction between the categories tends to blur. Some people come for all three reasons at once and some seem to come for no reason at all. The important thing, however, is that for whatever reason they come the principles they are taught remain the same.

In the following pages I hope to shed some light on the development, nature and application of Alexander's principles. The book begins with a brief account of Alexander's life as it relates to his discoveries. I then go on to describe these discoveries in detail. My aim in this is threefold. First, I want to let the reader see for himself the scientific nature of Alexander's explorations. In his introduction to Alexander's book *The Use of the Self*, Dewey wrote:

> Those who do not identify science with a parade of technical vocabulary will find in this account the essentials of scientific method in any field of inquiry. They will find a record of long, continued, patient, unwearied experimentation and observation in which every inference is extended, tested, corrected by further more searching experiments. Personally, I cannot speak with too much admiration – in the original sense of wonder as well as the sense of respect – of the persistence and thoroughness with which these extremely difficult observations and experiments were carried out.[5]

And in his introduction to Alexander's *Constructive Conscious Control* Dewey added:

> After studying Mr. Alexander's method in actual operation, I would stake myself upon the fact that he has applied to our ideas and beliefs about ourselves and about our acts exactly the same method of experimentation and of production of new sensory observations, as tests and means of developing thought, that have been the source of all progress in the physical sciences.[6]

More recently, Professor Nikolaas Tinbergen, the 1973 Nobel Laureate in Medicine, has said, 'This story of perceptiveness, of intelligence, and of persistence shown by a man without medical training, is one of the true epics of medical research and practice.'[7]

The second reason for examining Alexander's process of discovery in detail is that the method he followed exemplifies exactly what his Technique cultivates – a 'questing' state of mind predicated on a commitment to taking responsibility for oneself. Alexander liked to say, 'You can do as I do if you do what I did.' No one, to my knowledge, has done what he did. We can, however, learn from his example, so long as we keep in mind Aldous Huxley's statement that, even with the help of an Alexander teacher, 'one has to make the discovery oneself, starting from scratch.'

Third, I want to give the reader a clear picture of what I consider to be the basic operational ideas used in teaching and learning Alexander's methods. In Part 2, I discuss each of these ideas in some detail, relating them to my own experience and showing how they arose from Alexander's practical work and were not merely the product of theory. Although the Alexander lesson of today differs from Alexander's original experiments, the essence remains the same. In Part 3, I discuss the importance of the Technique in learning how to learn and show its relevance to the education of children.

This is not intended to be the ultimate work on the Alexander Technique but rather a simple introduction to the subject based on my own experience of applying the Technique in everyday life. Indeed it would be unwise to attempt much more, for what we are considering is not a final, perfected theory. In Alexander's own words: 'We are only at the beginning of understanding.'

1

The Man
and His
Discovery

*'He who knows that power is
inborn... and so perceiving,
throws himself unhesitatingly
on his thought, instantly rights
himself, stands in the erect
position, commands his limbs,
works miracles.'*

RALPH WALDO EMERSON

Alexander:
the man
and his
discovery

Frederick Matthias Alexander was born at Wynyard on the north-west coast of Tasmania, Australia, in 1869, the oldest of eight children. He was brought up on a large, isolated farm where self-sufficiency was not an abstract concept: when the roof leaked, one fixed it or got wet. Alexander was a precocious child and, suffering from recurring respiratory difficulties, was taken out of school to be educated privately. As his health began to improve from about the age of nine, he developed a passion for horses and gradually became expert at training and managing them. His other great love was the theatre, particularly Shakespeare, and throughout his life he kept up an active enthusiasm for these two very different interests.

At the age of sixteen financial pressures forced him to leave the country life he loved for the mining town of Mount Bischoff. During the day he worked at a variety of jobs and in the evenings he studied music and drama and taught himself the violin. After three years he moved to Melbourne, where he continued his dramatic and musical training under the best teachers, visiting theatres, concerts and art galleries and organizing his own amateur dramatic company in his spare time. When his money ran out, he took odd jobs as a clerk or an accountant, even working as a tea-taster on one occasion. However, recurrent illness

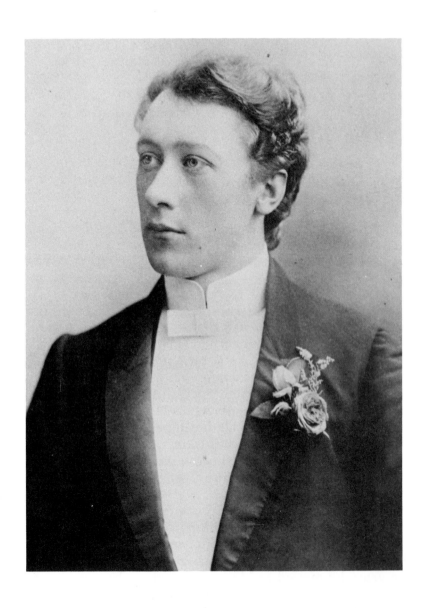

F.M. Alexander as a young man: a portrait taken for his theatrical portfolio.

and what was then a violent temper, along with a distaste for commercial life, ensured that he never held any job for very long. In his early twenties, he decided to devote himself to a career as an actor and reciter, and he soon established an excellent reputation, giving recitals, concerts and private engagements and producing plays. His speciality was a one-man show of dramatic and humorous pieces heavily laced with Shakespeare.

There was only one cloud on the horizon: a persistent tendency to hoarseness and respiratory trouble that affected the quality of his voice during recitations. Voice teachers and medical men advised rest, and Alexander found that the symptoms disappeared so long as he did not attempt to recite. On one occasion he rested his voice for two weeks before a particularly important performance. Half-way through the show, it failed. Confronting his doctor, Alexander was told only that he should continue to rest his voice. Not being one to stand under a leaky roof, he decided to take matters into his own hands and to seek his own cure.

Clearly, something he was doing while using his voice was the source of the problem. As he had no apparent difficulties in ordinary speech, Alexander deduced that it must be something he was doing while reciting that was the cause of the problem. Standing in front of a mirror, he started to observe exactly what he called his 'manner of doing' – first while speaking and then, since he found nothing unusual, while reciting. As he started to recite he noticed three things: he stiffened his neck, so causing his head to retract (he later called this 'pulling the head back'); he depressed his larynx unduly; and he sucked in breath with a gasp. In more difficult passages the pattern became exaggerated. He soon realized that this pattern was also present in his ordinary speech, although it was so slight as to be barely noticeable, and that this meant that the difference between speaking and reciting was one of degree only.

Reasoning that the pattern must constitute a misuse since it seemed to be responsible for his problem, Alexander set out to try to prevent it. Although he could not stop himself depressing his larynx or gasping for breath by direct, conscious effort, he did at least partially succeed in preventing himself pulling back his head. What is more, this led to the disappearance of the other two harmful tendencies. As he got better at preventing this pattern of misuse, Alexander discovered that the quality of his voice improved, and his medical advisers also confirmed that his larynx was in a better condition.

From all this Alexander concluded that his 'manner of doing' did indeed affect his functioning. This was the beginning of his realization that the choices we make about what we do with ourselves to a large extent determine the quality of our lives. He called this power of choice 'Use'.

In an attempt to improve his functioning further, Alexander now started experimenting by putting his head forward. He observed, however, that when it passed a certain point he depressed his larynx, with the same effect as before. Seeking next a way of using his head and neck that did not involve depressing his larynx, he discovered that when he depressed his larynx he also tended to lift his chest, narrow his back and shorten his stature.

This observation was a turning-point. Alexander now understood that the functioning of his vocal mechanism was influenced not only by his head and neck but by the pattern of tension throughout his body. His next step was to prevent himself shortening his stature while maintaining the improved Use of his head and neck. His experiments showed that his voice functioned best when his stature lengthened and that this could only be achieved when he used his head in a way that he described as 'forward and up' in relation to his neck and torso. From this came his later discovery that the dynamic relationship of the head, neck and torso is the primary factor in organizing human movement, a special relationship that he termed the Primary Control.

Having reasoned out the steps to his goal, Alexander was now confident that he could combine the necessary elements of 'prevention and doing' while he was reciting. Bringing two more mirrors into service, he was surprised to discover that:

...at the critical moment when I tried to combine the prevention of shortening with a positive attempt to *maintain a lengthening and speak at the same time,* I did not put my head forward and up as I intended, but actually put it back. Here then was startling proof that I was doing the opposite of what I believed I was doing and of what I had decided I ought to do.[8]

Reflecting on his experiments in the light of thirty-five years' teaching experience, Alexander added:

I was indeed suffering from a delusion that is practically universal, the delusion that because we are able to do what we 'will to do' in acts that are habitual and involve familiar sensory experiences, we shall be equally successful in doing what we 'will to do' in acts which are contrary to our habit and therefore involve sensory experiences that are unfamiliar.[9]

Alexander continued to experiment, observing himself standing, walking and gesturing. He already knew that the patterns of tension and malcoordination throughout his body all appeared to be 'synchronized' with the imbalance of his head on his neck. Going on to examine their relationship with his mental conceptions of his actions, he began to understand that the patterns of misuse were not simply physical. They involved the whole of his body and mind. From this realization he came to formulate the idea of psychophysical unity, a truly revolutionary idea that became the cornerstone of his work.

Opposed to Alexander's desire to use his mind and body in this new way was an overwhelming habitual pattern. This pattern was particularly powerful in Alexander's case because it had been specifically cultivated during his theatrical training, when he had learnt how to stand and walk on the stage. The stimulus to misuse himself, he realized, was much stronger than his ability to change, and he was forced to conclude that his approach to the problem of improving his Use had been misdirected and that he had never consciously thought through the way in which he directed his Use of himself. Like everyone else, he did what 'felt right' in accordance with habit. Now that he had observed that he pulled his head back and down when he felt he was putting it forward and up, he had to admit that his sense of what felt right was unreliable. This was a disturbing discovery. It compelled him to question all his basic assumptions and also seemed to reveal a new area for the study of human behaviour. 'Surely if it is possible for feeling to become untrustworthy as a means of direction,' he wrote, 'it should also be possible to make it trustworthy again.'[10]

Alexander now set himself to overcome his difficulties by fleeing himself from his dependence on what felt right and relying instead on conscious reasoning alone. As he knew his voice functioned best when his stature lengthened and also that any attempt to bring about such lengthening would be based on his untrustworthy sense of what felt right, he decided that the habitual pattern had to be stopped at its source. He therefore practised receiving a stimulus and refusing to do anything immediately in response. (He called this process 'inhibition'.) He then experimented by consciously willing the lengthening rather than by attempting to 'do' it directly. (This he called 'direction'.) Once again, however, at the 'critical moment' when he began to speak, he observed that his habitual direction dominated his reasoned intention. 'I could see it actually happening in the mirror,' he wrote.

Now he realized that he must spend time practising this conscious mode of direction and that any new Use of himself based on this practice would feel wrong according to his old sensory standard. As he practised, he came to understand that there was no clear dividing line between habit and reasoned direction and that he could not prevent the two overlapping. In order to allow his reasoned direction to dominate habit, Alexander concluded that he must give up all thought of the end for which he was working and focus instead on the steps leading to that end (the 'means-whereby').

Taking now the problem of speaking a sentence, Alexander worked out a plan. First, he would inhibit his immediate response to speak the sentence, thereby stopping at its source the habitual uncoordinated direction. Second, he would consciously practise projecting the directions necessary for his improved Use of himself. Specifically, he would think of letting his neck be free and his head go forward and up so as to allow his torso to lengthen and widen. Third, he would continue to project these directions until he was confident that he could maintain them while speaking the sentence. Fourth, at the moment when he decided to speak the sentence he would stop again and consciously reconsider his decision. In other words he would leave himself free to perform another action, such as lifting an arm, walking or simply remaining still, but whatever he chose to do he would continue to project the directions for the new pattern of Use.

It worked! By paying attention to the quality of his action rather than to his specific goal, Alexander began to free himself from his unreasoned control of his organism.

He outwitted his instinctive habitual direction and in the process developed a new method of learning based on psychophysical integrity.

Continued practice of the new technique had an exhilarating effect on Alexander's entire being. His breathing difficulties disappeared, and he moved with a new air of lightness and grace. His fame as an actor grew, and he became especially celebrated for his striking voice. Other actors and members of his audience flocked to him for lessons in voice production. Finding that words were insufficient to convey his experiences, he now began to devise a subtle process of manual guidance that would directly communicate the experience of improved psychophysical coordination, a process that he spent the rest of his life developing and refining.

Alexander's initial discoveries were made gradually over a period of years, during which he continued his stage career. His fame both as an actor and as a teacher grew, and by the mid-1890s he had a flourishing practice in Melbourne. At first his pupils came chiefly from the performing arts. As local doctors came to hear of his work, however, a few sent their patients to him, and before long these pupils outnumbered the ones with a theatrical background.

In 1899 Alexander moved to Sydney. His reputation preceded him, and he was soon inundated with work, although the medical establishment on the whole remained suspicious. One famous surgeon whom Alexander did win over was J.W. Steward McKay. The story goes that when they first met McKay remarked, 'If your teaching is sound, I'll make you, but if it's not I'll break

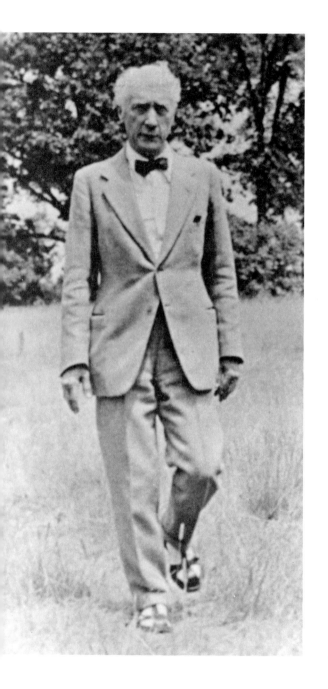

Even in the later years of his life, Alexander had a strong presence. In this photograph he is extremely alert, and yet his hands are relaxed and easy by his side. His movement is finely balanced and light.

you.' Alexander's response was characteristic. He shook McKay's hand warmly, saying, 'You are the man I have been looking for.' It was McKay who convinced him that he must move to London to gain the recognition his work deserved, and in April 1904 Alexander set sail, having first made an extensive farewell tour with *Hamlet* and *The Merchant of Venice* played by a company made up almost entirely of pupils who had been referred by doctors.

In London, Alexander's practice developed rapidly, and he soon became known as 'the protector of the London theatre'. Many of the most celebrated actors and actresses of the day took lessons from him, among them Sir Henry Irving, Matheson Lang, Oscar Asche, Lily Blayton and Viola and Beerbohm Tree. As his work became more widely known he had to deal with those who tried to copy and cheapen it. To forestall would-be plagiarists he published in 1910 his first book, *Man's Supreme Inheritance*, the theme of which he described as 'the great phase in Man's development when he passes from subconscious to conscious control of his mind and body'. The book was very well received and remained in print throughout Alexander's life.

The outbreak of war in 1914 brought an immediate decline in the number of pupils. Alexander knew that unless he could continue to teach he would lose the skills and understanding he had laboriously developed, and so he decided to move to the United States. In New York he knew just two people, but within a few weeks personal recommendations had brought him a teeming practice. For the next ten years he spent half the year in the United States and half in Britain, taking on an assistant in each country to cope with the demand for lessons.

Between the two world wars Alexander's work continued to expand and flourish. He had a substantial teaching practice and gained a number of influential supporters, among them William Temple, Archbishop of Canterbury, Sir Stafford Cripps, Esther Lawrence of the Froebel Institute, George Bernard Shaw and Aldous Huxley. In 1923 Alexander's second book, *Constructive Conscious Control of the Individual*, was published, with a foreword by John Dewey, the American educational philosopher who became one of the most ardent and consistent advocates of the

Alexander Technique. Dewey wrote that Alexander's work contained 'the promise and potentiality of the new direction that is needed in all education'. Like Dewey, Alexander believed that education was the key to social evolution and in 1924 he established at his studio in London the first school to be based on his principles. Run by Irene Tasker, a fully qualified teacher who had trained with Montessori, it took children aged between three and eight; although a conventional infants' school curriculum was followed, the main emphasis was on teaching the children a proper Use of themselves. After ten years, Tasker emigrated to South Africa, where she became the first Alexander teacher to set up an independent practice, and the school moved from London to the country under the direction of Margaret Goldie. In 1940 it was evacuated to the United States, but attempts to re-establish it in England after the war failed.

For many years Alexander had been urged to set up a formal training course for potential teachers of the Technique. He held back, wanting to be sure there was sufficient demand for his work and, most important, to be certain that he could train his pupils to the highest standard. Would-be teachers of his work, he believed, had to be trained to put its principles and procedures into practice in their Use of themselves in daily activities before they could attempt to teach others to do likewise. Alexander's brother, Albert Redden (A.R.), had already shown the success of Alexander's teaching methods. After crushing his spine in a riding accident, A.R. had been told that he would never walk again. He spent his convalescence on his back, practising the processes of inhibition and conscious direction. Within eighteen months he had recovered, and he continued to teach the Technique until his death in 1947. With his brother's example in mind, Alexander eventually inaugurated the three-year Training Course for Teachers in 1930.

Alexander's third book, *The Use of the Self*, in which he set out to describe the process by which he worked out the Technique, was first published in 1932. Nine years later came his final book, *The Universal Constant in Living*. This consisted of a collection of articles on the concept of Use in which Alexander laid particular stress on the harmful effects of 'physical culture' and exercise systems that ignored the unity of mind and body. Shortly after the end of the war, Alexander's supporters in South Africa attempted to replace the methods of physical education practised there with a system based on Alexander's ideas. This led to a venomous attack on Alexander and his work by Dr Ernst Jokl, director of the South African Physical Education Committee. Having exhausted diplomatic channels in an attempt to clear his name, Alexander sued for libel. In a bitterly contested case that lasted four years, Alexander found many medical men ranged against him. Two extremely influential men did declare for Alexander, however, testifying to the scientific validity of his work. These were Sir Charles Sherrington, the Nobel prize-winning neurophysiologist, and Professor Raymond Dart, the great anthropologist.

Alexander eventually won the case in 1948, although a severe stroke which paralysed the left side of his body meant that he was unable to attend the trial. Applying the principles he had developed, Alexander fought his way to recovery. Now an old man, deprived of most of his strength, he had to rely more than ever upon the power of pure direction, and pupils say that he did his best teaching during the five years before his death. In these years he continued to refine his method, at the same time maintaining his private practice and supervising the work of his assistant teachers. He died after a short illness on 10 October 1955.

As this brief biographical sketch has shown, Alexander's achievement was immense. He developed, on his own, an entirely new scientific method of examining and solving a particular problem and in so doing established a revolutionary way of looking at human functioning. Yet it must be recognized that, despite all this, and despite the work of his followers in the forty years since his death, his name is not as celebrated as his work undoubtedly merits. He must surely be counted as one of the most underrated men of the twentieth century.

There are two main reasons why this should be so. The first lies within Alexander's own character, the second within the nature of the established institutions of society. Alexander was certainly larger than life, a man whose faults were as exaggerated as his

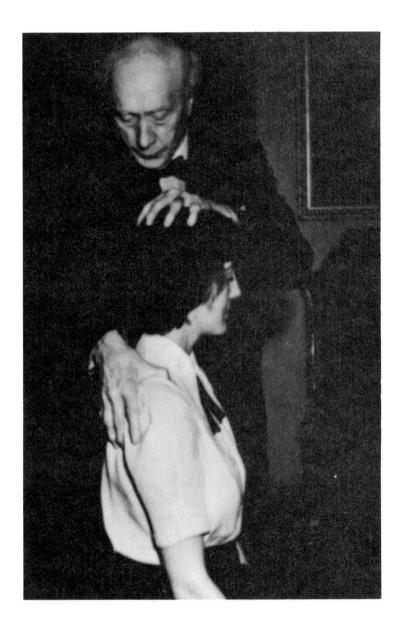

When working with a pupil Alexander was concerned with the total distribution of energy in the body throughout the lesson.

In this picture, with acute awareness of the information his hands and his eyes are giving him, he focuses on putting the pupil's body together so that she may experience a new dynamic relationship between all her body parts, especially her head, neck and upper back.

strengths. Those who knew him say that he was not the easiest of people to work with. He was not a sociable man and he was, above all, an individualist never content to fall in with the crowd. It may therefore be that his insistence on the highest standards, along with his understandable reluctance to entrust others with teaching the ideas he had so laboriously and painfully developed, led him, perhaps unconsciously, to avoid possibilities of publicizing the Technique. Certainly the number of teachers he trained was minute, too small to make a significant impression at any one time. It has only been during the last twenty years that a substantial number of teachers have completed their training and set up in practice and that the general public has in consequence begun to become familiar with the Technique.

It may be too that Alexander's very certainty about the Technique, the fact that he *knew* and was unwilling to waste time explaining and proving what he knew, served to discourage potential advocates. As George Bernard Shaw once remarked, 'Alexander calls upon the world to witness a change so small and subtle that only he can see it.' If people could not witness the change that Alexander had seen, and were unwilling to submit themselves to his methods, they had little alternative but to turn away without understanding.

Much the most important explanation of why Alexander's work lacked general acceptance lies in the fact that it was – and to a great extent still is – decades ahead of its time. It is not specifically medical, nor is it educational in the usual sense of that word; practitioners of these disciplines cannot readily and easily assimilate it and adapt it to their methods. The Technique demands a fundamental revision in the way an individual thinks about himself, and if it is to be accepted within society an even more fundamental collective revision of attitudes, by doctors, psychologists and teachers among many others, will be necessary.

2

The
Operational
Ideas

When an investigation comes to
be made, it will be found that
every single thing we are doing
in the work is exactly what is
being done in Nature where
the conditions are right, the
difference being that we
are learning to do
it consciously.

F.M. ALEXANDER

Alexander developed his ideas over a period of more than sixty years. As his teaching experience grew he expanded and refined the theoretical framework for his Technique. His theories on the corrupting factors in civilization and the evolution of consciousness are instructive, but the main thrust of his work was always practical and down-to-earth. In effect there are seven basic ideas which form the core of his teaching. I have called these 'operational ideas' because they serve as a useful guide to anyone who wishes to apply the Technique in daily life.

The operational ideas are:

Use and functioning
The whole person
Primary Control
Unreliable sensory appreciation
Inhibition
Direction
Ends and means

Let's consider them 'all together, one after the other...'.

Use and
functioning

*The most valuable knowledge we can possess
is of the use and functioning of the self.*

In *The Universal Constant in Living*, Alexander begins: 'Few of us, hitherto, have given consideration to the question of the extent to which we are individually responsible for the ills our flesh is heir to.' The question of individual responsibility is at the heart of Alexander's work. He realized that he had never taken responsibility for the direction of his Use of himself. Instead of employing his power of choice fully, he had always done what felt right. He had never questioned his unreasoned Use until he discovered that certain habits were interfering with his functioning. Then, when he did decide to exercise his power of choice, he came up against the almost overwhelming force of habit.

Commenting on this discovery, Walter Carrington wrote:

Alexander's experiments led him to study processes, of the nature of which he knew very little and, indeed, of which very little is still known by anybody. Even today, the human organism as a whole is largely unknown territory so far as experimental observation is concerned. The nature of the relationship between mind and body is still undetermined. The precise relationship between what we call the voluntary and the involuntary aspects of human behaviour is still unknown; and although we know a great deal more than was known in Alexander's early days about the structure and functioning of the nervous system, the exact nature of the processes of willing and wishing, of choice and selection of response, of thinking and feeling, and all the other so-called mental processes of which we are subjectively aware, is still largely a mystery.

It was this realization that led Alexander to choose terms for his descriptive needs that were at once as simple and as non-committal as possible. He saw that the borderline between the voluntary and the involuntary was too blurred to be capable of sharp distinction.[11]

Yet Alexander found he could make some choices, such as to speak or not to speak. This power of choice allowed him to determine, to a degree, the quality of the actions he chose. He came to understand that his power had much more potential than he was using at that time. His chapter on 'The Evolution of a Technique' in *The Use of the Self* recounts his attempts to take full command of his power to choose. He realized that the choices he made about the Use of his organism were fundamental, since they directly affected his functioning and therefore influenced all his other choices. Alexander employed the word Use to describe the process of control over all those actions that he seemed to have the potential to control.

The concept of Use has the same fundamental importance as 'heredity' and 'environment'. Heredity is usually considered to be the factor that sets our potential, environment the factor that determines the extent to which we actualize it. Use is necessary to complete the picture. Take the case of a man who drinks too much. His problem may result from a variety of hereditary and environmental influences. Eventually he perceives that his drinking is having a harmful effect, and he may therefore decide to stop. Although it may seem impossible for him simply to choose not to drink, the potential for that choice is there. Help may be sought through hypnosis, chemotherapy, psychoanalysis or voluntary incarceration. It is interesting, however, that the most successful form of treatment, that provided by Alcoholics Anonymous, sets out to put an individual in touch with his own sense of responsibility and integrity and to give him enough support to enable him to face facts and use his power of choice.

Alexander called this power of choice 'Man's Supreme Inheritance', perceiving that the way in which we use it affects our functioning at all levels. He discovered that he could use himself in different ways and that some ways were better than others in terms of functioning. We all know that the way we use a tool determines its effectiveness. A chisel used as a screwdriver will not only be inefficient, it will also become damaged. The analogy with the way we use ourselves is limited because the self is such a complex tool. Nevertheless, we do use ourselves for better or worse, consciously or unconsciously, all the time.

The effects of faulty Use tend to be overlooked. This is because on the whole bad Use does not have immediately observable serious consequences. It is like the continual dripping of water that wears away a stone. In *The Universal Constant in Living* Alexander states:

> A good manner of use of the self exerts an influence for good upon general functioning which is not only continuous, but also grows stronger as time goes on, becoming, that is, a *constant* influence tending always to raise the standard of functioning and improve the manner of reaction. A bad manner of use, on the other hand, continuously exerts an influence for ill, tending to lower the standard of general functioning, thus becoming a *constant* influence tending always to interfere with every functional activity arising from our response to stimuli from within and without the self, and harmfully affecting the manner of every reaction.[12]

It is interesting to note that those most frequently seeking Alexander lessons have always been musicians, actors and dancers, whose quality of Use directly affects their ability to make a living.

Since Use influences different levels of functioning, the physical, emotional and mental, let us consider the effects of the Alexander Technique on this relationship. This separation of the different levels is for purposes of analysis only – in practice we always use ourselves as a whole.

The effect of bad Use on our physical condition is the easiest to observe. Doctors have been aware for many years of a range of

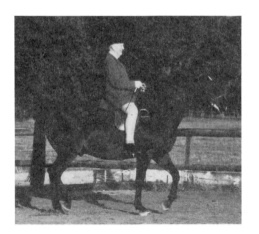

USE AFFECTS FUNCTION

In all activities our Use affects our functioning. A rider's Use affects his own functioning and that of the horse as well. Walter Carrington demonstrates poise on horseback.

Maintaining good Use while learning enhances our ability to learn. Responses and reflexes become more accurate, stress is minimized and an alert quietness allows the absorption of new material.

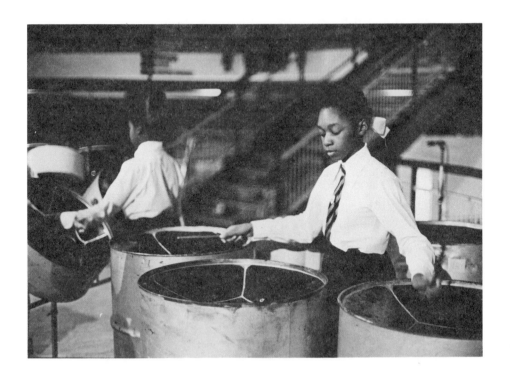

diseases that often seem not to have organic causes. Examples include the proverbial bad back, headaches, fatigue and asthma. These are called 'functional disorders' or 'psychosomatic problems' and doctors generally treat them with a variety of palliative measures. If these do not work the patient is usually referred to a psychiatrist.

In his classic study *Body Mechanics,* Dr J.E. Goldthwaite presents dramatic photographs of the compression and congestion to which internal organs are exposed as the result of poor body Use. They show how the inefficiency with which we use our bodies takes its toll, interfering with breathing and compressing unduly the joints and internal organs.

Dr Wilfred Barlow, a well-known physician and teacher of the Alexander Technique, has found that misuse is usually a major factor in both causing and perpetuating rheumatism, backache, arthritis, breathing disorders, hypertension, fatigue, gastro-intestinal conditions, headaches and certain sexual problems. He reports success in treating all these through re-educating his patients by means of the Alexander Technique. His treatment is always directed towards Use as a whole and not towards a specific symptom. Barlow also emphasizes the importance of the Alexander Technique in replacing the traditional medical orientation towards curing disease with a preventive approach.

Many other physicians have recognized the value of the Alexander Technique in preventing and treating disease. In a letter written to the *British Medical Journal* in 1936, nineteen prominent British doctors testified that they had observed consistent improvements in patients referred for Alexander lessons, even in cases of chronic disease. They emphasized that misuse was a major factor in causing disease and that diagnosis of a patient therefore remained incomplete unless it took into account the influence of Use upon functioning. More recently, Alexander's teaching has received support from Dr John Diamond, President of the International Academy of Preventive Medicine, Drs Garlick, Libet, Austin and Somner, and from Nikolaas Tinbergen.

To put it simply, bad body Use results in unbalanced coordination; some parts of the body do too much work, others do too little. A classic example is lifting. Most people tend to overtense their arms, shoulders and necks while collapsing their backs and stiffening their legs.

Tonight when you brush your teeth, or the next time you pick up a pen to write, observe the way you distribute your energy. Is it really necessary to tense your neck and interfere with your breathing in order to do these things? If you do not notice anything unusual, you should refer to the chapter on Unreliable Sensory Appreciation on page 52.

All this may not seem to be overwhelmingly important. But it is worth bearing in mind the words of the philosopher Herbert Spencer:

> Each faculty acquires fitness for its function by performing its function; and if its function is performed for it by a substitute agency, none of the required adjustment of nature takes place, but the nature becomes deformed to fit the artificial arrangements instead of the natural arrangements.[13]

Over the years my attempts to refine my own Use have resulted in improvements in both functioning and structure. After my first few Alexander lessons it became obvious that I was employing 'artificial arrangements' in my movement. For instance, when I bent down I tended to stiffen my knees and break at the waist instead of using my hip and knee joints properly. At the same time I found that the stiffening of my knees was causing me to hold my breath and that my lumbar vertebrae were displaced at precisely the point from which I bent. This was just one aspect of a pattern of misuse that not only had a detrimental effect on my functioning but also distorted my structure – and it was a revelation to discover where my joints really were and how they were meant to work in relation to one another. Now my general health and vitality have increased and I have become completely free of backache and stiff neck. I have gained half an inch in height and greater fullness in my back, and in addition I experience a growing sense of freedom and a joy of movement in all activities.

Improved vitality and health will obviously have positive effects on emotional life. However, the importance of Use in emotional functioning goes much deeper than this. Writing about

Alexander's work, Aldous Huxley said, 'If you teach an individual first to be aware of his physical organism and then to use it as it was meant to be used you can often change his entire attitude to life and cure his neurotic tendencies.' Huxley's statement is based in part on the assumption articulated by Dewey that 'all of the psychic complexes have their basis in organic discoordinations and tensions with compensatory flabbiness.' The important thing to understand about this last statement is that specific 'discoordinations and tensions' are inseparable parts of a whole pattern.

This pattern is the result of two major factors. The first, which was first described by Wilhelm Reich, concerns the relationship of emotional upheaval and trauma, particularly in early childhood, with the formation of 'energy blocks' and 'character armouring'. In other words, our reaction to disturbing events throws our bodies into chronic imbalance. We tend to hold the 'memory' of a traumatic experience in a particular part of the body. This muscular memory in time becomes part of the total pattern and is incorporated into an individual's Use of himself. Failure to take responsibility for one's Use assures that the memory remains.

The other factor has been pointed out by Dr Barlow in *The Alexander Principle*. He wrote that 'Many habitual postures do not represent an immediate expression of an emotion but are rather a position from which certain actions and emotions can be possible.' In other words certain emotions such as joy or depression are only possible with certain configurations of musculature. Barlow goes on to say that these configurations do not necessarily start as overtly emotional responses, but, for example, from the way we use our bodies in recurrent work situations:

> The office worker, the conveyor belt engineer, the lorry driver, the mum-bent-over-baby, the dentist, the pianist, carry out occupations for so long that they eventually will hold themselves partially contracted even when they are not involved in the actual pressures of their jobs. This residual tension may not be conscious but eventually it is maintained most of the time. The summation of their various temporary attitudes

31

eventually finds its expression in a posture – or in a limited repertoire of postures, which come to dominate a person's character. In small and at first unobtrusive ways we become enslaved to our past.[14]

My work with the Alexander Technique has helped me become aware of my 'repertoire' of posture and habit and of the associated emotional patterns. I have learnt what I do with myself when I am depressed, afraid, nervous, insincere, happy, attentive and so on. Each of these states has a characteristic postural manifestation. As I have become more familiar with the subtleties of the different patterns I find myself freer to change stereotyped and immature behaviour. These patterns represent one's character. I used to be 'characterized' by a raised chest, tight stomach, set jaw and hunched shoulders – the classic male defensive–aggressive posture. Now I am free to save this for special occasions!

The Alexander Technique involves an ever-deepening process of discovery and change, a process that works gently but powerfully. Its dynamics have been well expressed by Frank Jones:

> The changes I observed in myself were often unexpected, but they were never accompanied by any sudden or violent release of emotion and never left me feeling defenceless. The Alexander Technique provides the knowledge and freedom to change, but it is change within a developmental model. There is no 'must'. Changes take place when you are ready for them and can permit them to happen. Habitual tensions that have grown up over a long time limit development and prevent the free expression of personality. They serve as protection, however, in situations where, rightly or wrongly, a person feels vulnerable or incompetent. The Alexander Technique does not deprive one of this 'character armouring' as long as it is needed. Lessons in the Technique release an organic process of change that gradually replaces old habits with new habits which are flexible and can themselves be changed. The process of change is not mindless. It can be directed by intelligence into paths that lead to the best development of the individual's own personality.[15]

As one of my colleagues put it, 'The Alexander Technique always uncovers the cracks behind the wallpaper; but it only does so when the person has enough new plaster to refill them!'

Dewey believed that the Technique was a method of enlightening the emotions. At the intellectual level, according to Jones:

> [Dewey] found it much easier, after he had studied the Technique, to hold a philosophical position calmly once he had taken it or to change it if new evidence came up warranting a change. He contrasted his own attitude with the rigidity of other academic thinkers who adopt a position early in their career and then use their intellects to defend it indefinitely.[16]

Dewey believed that the formation and execution of ideas depended on habit. 'Reason pure of all influence from prior habit is fiction,' he said, adding that 'the real opposition is not between reason and habit, but between routine unintelligent habit and intelligent habit or art.'[17]

We must have creative and adaptable habits in order to cope with our complex world. The key function of the intellect is to monitor the effectiveness of habit and determine where changes should be made. It can be compared with the role of a good industrial manager who monitors and directs his subordinates without trying to do their work for them.

Intelligence must be balanced with our other functions. In our culture many individuals live 'in their heads'. (Dewey, in his pre-Alexander days, was a prime example.) The development of mind–body coordination which comes through improved Use creates a practical framework in which the intelligence can work. In this way our intellects can become competent servants rather than incompetent masters.

The organization of our physical, emotional and intellectual functions is extremely complex. The important thing to remember about these three functions is that we do have a choice about the way we employ them. *The most fundamental form of misuse is the failure to make choices.* We can choose to have a choice! One criterion that we must employ in making these choices is the effect they will have on our functioning. One of the goals of the Alexander Technique is to create the conditions necessary for 'natural functioning' through a balanced distribution of energy, each part of the system performing its own work in harmony with the rest. This is the true meaning of 'poise'. The body is our instrument for fulfilling our purpose on earth. This instrument can be coarse and dull or finely tuned and receptive – the choice is ours.

Checkpoints

How does your Use of yourself affect your functioning?

Are you aware of your habits of moving, thinking and feeling? Try listing three habits of body use, thought or emotion.

Have you ever successfully changed a habit? How did you do it?

How has your character been influenced by your heredity? your environment? your Use?

The whole
person

*...the so-called 'mental' and 'physical' are not
separate entities... all training... must be based
on the indivisible unity of the human organism.*

The threefold model of human functioning referred to in the previous chapter (page 25) is a useful tool for understanding many of our personal difficulties, so long as we keep in mind that the whole is more than the sum of its parts. Most personality problems are the result of conflict between these parts. Our bodies tell us one thing, our thoughts another and our emotions yet another (for example, I want to eat some cake; no, I shouldn't, I'll get fat; I feel guilty about eating, and so on).

This simplification expresses what I call the individual mind–body problem. We often behave as though we were not one whole system but a compilation of different little personalities. Just as our necks and shoulders often do the work of our backs, so our emotions often do the work of our intellects, and vice versa. This uneconomical use of energy creates inner conflict and can obscure an individual's sense of identity.

Such lack of inner harmony does not appear surprising when we look at the nature of the institutions that dominate our society. In Dewey's words, 'The world seems mad in preoccupation with what is specific, particular and disconnected in medicine, politics, science, industry and education.'[18]

In medicine, for example, treatment is all too often of individual parts rather than of the whole. In recent years, doctors have tended to specialize more and more, and general practice has

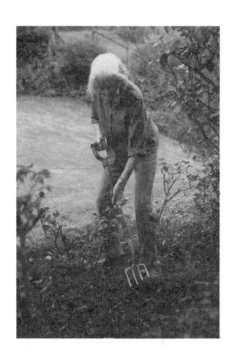

THE WHOLE PERSON

A healthy person with a harmonious relationship between mind, emotions and body will exude a sense of well-being.

The appearance of 80-year-old Chile Eagar, who trained with Alexander himself, conveys to us the qualities in her character. At this age, her body is formed into the shape of her underlying traits and attitudes, conveying dignity, alertness and presence.

The two young women communicate a sense of wholeness and ease. One can imagine them entering freely into any of the basic emotional states – joy, fear, sadness, anger, reverence – as their bodies do not show a holding of any one pattern of emotional response.

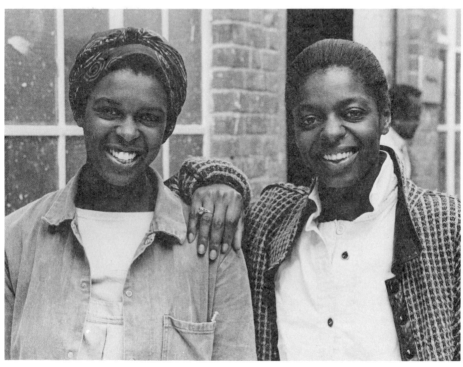

come to be seen as a relatively unglamorous form of medical care. This can mean that a particular consultant will know all about your eyes, say, or your ears, nose and throat, a great deal about the rest of you, and hardly anything at all about your total condition. Western medicine concentrates more on the direct alleviation of specific symptoms than on the underlying causes that may provoke them. New and more powerful drugs are constantly being developed in an attempt to suppress the manifestations of disease. To a certain extent these drugs do succeed, but at the same time they often create increasingly resilient viral and bacterial strains as well as a wide range of side effects, some of which, as in the case of thalidomide, can be horrifying. On a less dramatic level the widespread use of painkillers, tranquillizers and other everyday drugs reflects our inability to get to the source of our problems.

This 'disconnected' approach is also evident in our educational system which still over-emphasizes examination results at the expense of real learning. Our children are fed vast quantities of discrete and often unrelated information which they must parrot back on demand. They are drilled and judged on their performance in a series of disconnected topics. Physical education is usually seen as just another 'subject', quite separate and not as important as the traditional three Rs. Indeed, the very term 'physical education' suggests the belief that the mind and the body can be educated separately.

Seeing these imbalances, many people have recognized and come to understand the need for wholeness. They have realized that the starting-point is the individual himself or herself. The tremendous popularity of Eastern philosophy and Western psychotherapy is evidence of this. But how are we to avoid approaching these disciplines in the same disconnected manner in which we have been schooled, 'cured' and processed? Professor Dewey understood this problem when he wrote in his introduction to *Man's Supreme Inheritance*:

When the organs through which any structure, be it physiological, mental or social, are out of balance, when they are uncoordinated, specific and limited attempts at a cure only exercise the disordered mechanism. In 'improving' one organic structure they produce a compensatory maladjustment somewhere else.

Clearly, we must find a balanced way through which we can approach ourselves. The advantage of Alexander's work is that his idea of psychophysical unity is not just theoretical, it is the product of his own experience of wholeness. When he began the process that led to his discovery he believed, like most other people, that 'mind' and 'body' were separate entities. Experience soon revealed that this was not so. First he realized that his voice problem was not the result merely of the misuse of his vocal mechanism but was caused by a response of his whole body. Later he found that every idea, such as to 'speak a sentence', was inevitably associated with a response of his whole body. These discoveries about himself were confirmed by his teaching experience, and he became convinced that the so-called 'mental' and 'physical' could not be divorced from one another and that human ills and shortcomings could not be so classified and then dealt with accordingly. He argued that all training, of whatever kind, must be based on the understanding that the human organism always functions as a whole and can only be changed *fundamentally* as a whole.

A practical understanding of the idea of psychophysical unity is not easy to come by. People often come to Alexander lessons

THIS IS MY HEAD.   IT THINKS. IT TALKS. IT CHARMS.   IT WORRIES. IT LAUGHS. IT HURTS.   IT HAS A HUNDRED WONDERFUL TRICKS.   I AM PROUD OF IT.   THIS IS MY BODY

because of a 'bad back' or some other symptom. They are surprised to find that they are not asked to take off their clothes for an examination and that a diagnosis of their complaint will not be offered. Others who may have an emotional problem are equally surprised to find that the focus of lessons is not on analysing trauma, 'character armour' or past events. New pupils also tend to ask for exercises that will bring about the experience they get in lessons. It is a while before they understand that until a new coordination is learned any exercise will simply mean practising their bad habits. If an individual has a tendency to stiffen his neck and discoordinate himself every time he makes a single movement, then he will stiffen his neck and discoordinate himself even more when he tries to do an exercise.

When an Alexander teacher puts her hand on a pupil, she gets a sense of that person's potential for coordinating the whole of himself. She does not attempt to fix a stiff shoulder or hip but rather to teach her pupil to integrate these parts into a functional unity. Nor does she try to cure a depression but rather to teach her pupil how to use himself in such a way as to prevent him depressing himself further.

I now realize that when I first came to take Alexander lessons, I shared all these misconceptions, although at the same time I professed a belief, based mainly on theoretical considerations, in the unity of mind and body. It was not until I had studied the Technique for some time that this belief became a practical real-

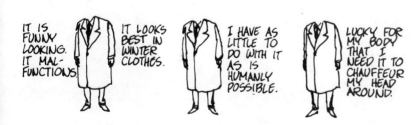

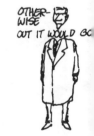

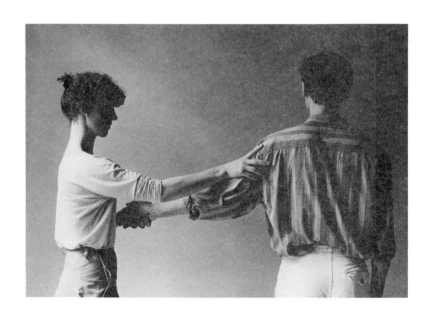

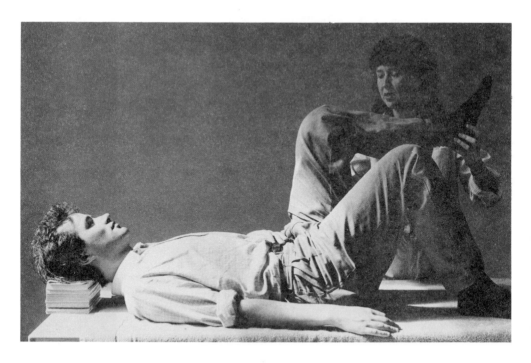

In an Alexander lesson the limbs are guided in such a way as to increase their connection with the torso while leaving the fundamental balance of the head, neck and back undisturbed. The muscle groups within the limbs are encouraged to release to their full resting length. As a result the pupil experiences improved coordination and a corresponding sense of expansion and aliveness.

ity for me. My own discovery to some extent paralleled Alexander's. First I became tangibly aware that my body functioned as a whole. An experience in one of my earliest lessons did much to make me understand this. The teacher had his hand on the back of my neck and asked me to release the undue tension I had created in my right ankle. I had the strong impression that he could feel all the tensions in my body, that he knew me better than I myself did. When I did release my right ankle I was suddenly able to feel a connection between my neck and foot that I had never felt before. Then, as I experienced more of these connections, I began to become aware of what I was doing with myself to create disconnections. I discovered that what I was doing was not just something physical but was mental and emotional as well. In other words, I experienced the unity of these elements in action. My greatest insight came after one lesson in which I had a sense of being completely connected in body and mind. There I was, and that was it – there were no more separate elements. Although the effect eventually wore off, I had been given a taste of what my full potential might be.

Checkpoints

What does wholeness mean to you? Express your concept of wholeness in writing, drawing or through some other creative means.

Do you ever experience conflicts between different parts of your self? Describe them, then try diagramming them.

In your daily life, when do you experience wholeness? disconnection? Describe the difference.

41

Primary
control

*... there is a primary control of the use of the
self, which governs the working of all the
mechanisms, and so renders the control of the
complex human organism relatively simple.*

In *The Endeavour of Jean Fernel* Sir Charles Sherrington writes:

> Mr Alexander has done a service to the study of man by insis-
> tently treating each act as involving the whole integrated indi-
> vidual, the whole psychophysical man. To take a step is an
> affair, not of this or that limb solely, but of the total neuro-
> muscular activity of the movement – not least of the head and
> neck.[19]

Indeed, not least of the head and neck. Alexander first of all
discovered that the relationship of his head and neck had immediate consequences for the condition of his larynx and breathing mechanism and then that the Use of his head and neck was
the prime factor in coordinating the Use of the rest of his organism. He functioned best when his stature lengthened, and this
came about when he allowed a Use of his head that he described
as 'forward and up' in relation to his neck and torso. The reader
will recall that when Alexander first tried to 'put' his head
forward and up he found that he could not do so. Eventually he
realized that to achieve his goal he should not 'do' or 'put'
anything, but rather apply a process of noninterfering (inhibition) and conscious reasoned intention (direction).

In other words, Alexander's experience taught him that
the relationship of the head, neck and torso was of primary

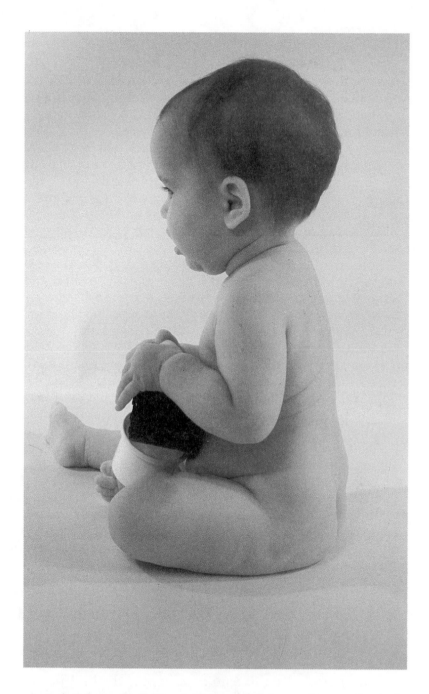

An infant keeps its head poised through balance, the muscles in its back supporting the spine perfectly erect. There is no tension in the neck muscles, and no sense of the fatigue that adults associate with sitting up straight.

importance in determining his level of functioning and in organizing his reactions into a coordinated whole. He coined the phrase 'Primary Control' to indicate this relationship.

Alexander has often been misinterpreted as advocating a 'right position' for the head, and 'Primary Control' has been misunderstood to suggest a specific anatomical centre or magic button. This is simply not so. The Primary Control is a dynamic, ever-changing *relationship* that functions all the time, for better or worse, in every position. Yet some positions of the body are obviously better than others, in terms of both their practical efficiency and their effect on functioning. Alexander called these 'positions of mechanical advantage'. The main concern of the Alexander Technique, however, is not to teach better positions but to teach the better Use of ourselves that results in better positions.

The right working of the Primary Control can best be seen in the movements of animals, infants and a few outstanding adults. My favourite examples include Muhammad Ali in his prime, Artur Rubinstein and Fred Astaire. These people display grace and ease in their every movement. Compare the poised relationship of their head, neck and torso with that of people one sees on the train or in the bar or with a classic example of bad coordination such as the late Richard Nixon.

The head, neck and torso are linked in an extremely delicate and vulnerable postural relationship. The head, besides housing the brain, eyes, ears, nose and mouth, is also the locus of the two main balancing mechanisms, the optical and vestibular. The importance of the head's balance in relation to the rest of the body becomes even greater when looked at in the context of evolution. The upright posture is the result of millions of years of development and is the most advanced stage of the evolutionary process. It allows us the possibility of greater freedom and a better capacity for all-round movement than any other mammal. It extends our visual range and frees our upper limbs, making possible fine hand movements. It also increases our store of potential energy, allowing movements to be undertaken in the most economical way possible, so long as the balancing mechanism is not interfered with. And it promotes the best possible functioning of the body's life-support systems (i.e. breathing,

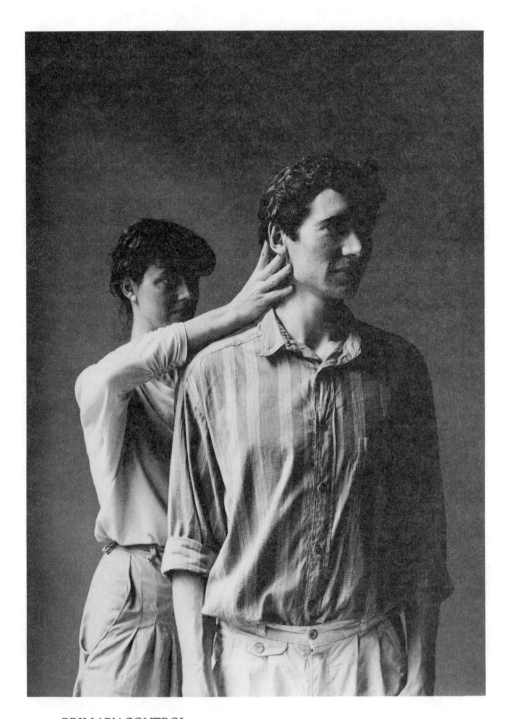

PRIMARY CONTROL
An Alexander teacher works with her pupil towards a free, dynamic
relationship between the head, neck and upper back.

circulation, digestion) and of the intelligence and emotions.

What kind of use do we make of this birthright? Professor Raymond Dart, an authority on anatomy, wrote that the condition of malposture was 'pandemic' in our urbanized culture.[20] Although most people seem to believe that they understand what proper posture is, they generally apologize for not having it themselves. The notion of posture tends to have negative associations with admonitions from school teachers and drill sergeants. Most of us take the whole question for granted.

Failure to adopt the fully upright posture represents a failure to explore our potential to be fully human. Unfortunately, we do not seem to be aware that we have a choice in the matter. In this connection Walter Carrington has written:

> The more we learn of how the organism works, the more we begin to appreciate its vast complexities, the more obvious it becomes that we cannot hope to achieve much by means of direct cortical intervention. (This is why admonitions are always hopeless.) The control that can be consciously exercised is a control of choice, a decision to act or not to act in a certain manner, in a certain direction, at a certain time.[21]

Sir Charles Sherrington puts it thus: 'The mastery of the brain over the reflex machinery does not take the form of inter-meddling with reflex details, rather, it dictates to a reflex mechanism "you may act" or "you may not act".'[22]

In trying to solve his voice problem, Alexander discovered that he could not get very far by 'direct cortical intervention' or by 'inter-meddling with reflex details' (i.e. by trying to *put* his head forward and up). Instead, he had to refine his power of choice so that he could effectively say 'you may act' to the reflex mechanism that allows the upright posture to be adopted fully. Dewey grasped the significance of this:

> This discovery corrects the ordinary conception of the conditioned reflex. The latter as usually understood renders an individual a passive puppet to be played upon by external manipulations. The discovery of a central control which condi-

tions all other reactions brings the conditioning factor under conscious direction and enables the individual through his own co-ordinated activities to take possession of his own potentialities.[23]

Research into animal behaviour has tended to support Alexander's ideas. George Coghill (1872–1941), a biologist who spent forty years studying animal development and behaviour, concluded that movement was controlled and integrated by the 'total pattern' of the head, neck and torso. This dominated the 'partial pattern' of the limbs. He wrote to Alexander, 'I am... amazed to see how you, years ago, discovered in human physiology and psychology the same principle which I worked out in the behaviour of lower vertebrates.' The biologist Rudolf Magnus (1873–1927) demonstrated that the head–neck–torso relationship was the *Zentralapparat* (central mechanism) in orienting an animal in its environment. He distinguished two basic and complementary forms of animal reactions which he called 'attitudinal' and 'righting' reflexes. When a cat sees a mouse it turns its head towards it and in a reflex action its body prepares itself to strike. This is the attitudinal reflex – it is as though the head of the cat imposed a specific attitude on the rest of its body. If the mouse crawls out of sight the cat returns to a balanced resting state, the dominant role in this righting reflex again being played by the head–neck–torso relationship. Magnus states that: 'It is possible to impress upon the whole body different adapted attitudes by changing only the position of the head.... The mechanism as a whole acts in such a way that the head leads and the body follows.[24]

Magnus himself made the comparison with human behaviour, emphasizing the importance of the righting reflexes in ensuring a return to a balanced resting state. 'In this way,' he added, 'all the senses of the body regain their precise relation to the outer world.' Magnus's research thus proposes another way of understanding misuse – in terms of interference with the reflex return to a balanced resting state – and suggests that the Alexander Technique can be understood as a means to free ourselves from habitual interference with our own 'righting reflexes'.

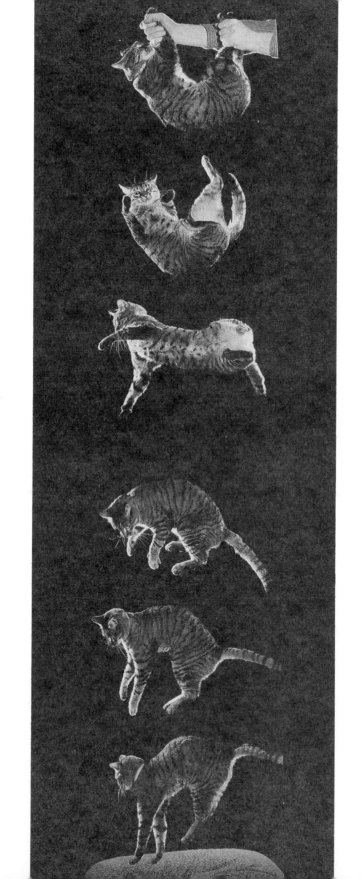

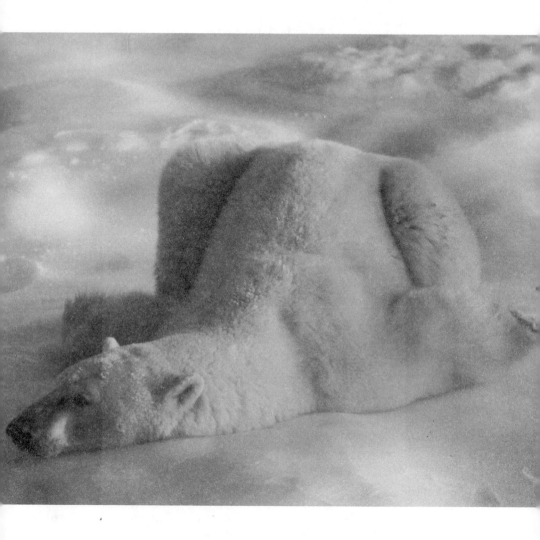

Organisms at all levels of evolutionary development, including humans, organize their movement by leading with the head and letting the body follow. This is easier to see in four-footed animals.

The falling cat provides a dramatic example of 'righting reflexes' in action. The eyes and head lead the body back to balance.

The polar bear offers a magnificent demonstration of the 'Balanced Resting State' (see page 161).

One of the aims of an Alexander lesson is to give the pupil the experience of a balanced working of the Primary Control. This is not an end in itself but rather a preparation for activity. I know from my own experience that when this balanced Use is maintained in movement the quality of action changes. Movement becomes lighter and easier, breathing becomes more rhythmic, and internal (proprioceptive) stimuli are perceived at the same time as external (perceptive) stimuli to create an integrated experience of the environment. In other words, you have a better sense of where you are (and sometimes even of who you are).

Frank Jones has produced experimental evidence supporting these claims. Employing multiple-image photography, electromyographic technique, X-ray photography and a strain-gauge platform, he has shown that the alteration of head balance achieved by applying the Alexander Technique results in a facilitation of what he calls the human 'antigravity system'. This system, which is made up of the spine, connective tissue and specialized muscles, and in effect serves to keep people upright, is essential to human life and functions all the time with varying degrees of efficiency.

The Alexander Technique encourages the lengthening of habitually contracted muscles of the spine, with the result that the upright posture is supported by a better balance of the skeletal and muscular system. This balance is reflected in improved muscle tone and a corresponding expansion in the spine. A key role in this expansion is played by the fluid-filled cartilaginous discs between the vertebrae. When the bones and muscles start to work in a balanced way, undue pressure on the discs is relieved and they can expand. This may be a major factor in producing the kinaesthetic experience of lightness and the increases in height that characterize the effects of the Technique.

Perhaps the most interesting aspect of Jones's work is his research into the 'startle pattern', a stereotyped response elicited by a sudden noise. The characteristic response starts with a disturbance of the head–neck–torso relationship, followed by a raising of the shoulders and a tensing of the chest and knees. All of this results in a loss of tone in the antigravity system. Jones reports that 'whenever the stimulus was strong enough to elicit a response, it appeared in the neck muscles and in many cases it appeared nowhere else.'[25]

Professor Dart has described the startle pattern as a prototypical response to fear. Jones, who calls it a paradigm for malposture, has shown that it varies very little from person to person and that it serves as a model for other, slower, response patterns. He points out that fear, anxiety, fatigue and pain all show postural deviations from the norm similar to those seen in the startle pattern. When one falls into a period of depression, pain or fear, the balance of the head, neck and torso is acutely disturbed. When the difficult period clears, one is often left with a habit of carrying the head in an unbalanced way. My own observations have convinced me that the majority of people spend much of their time in a modified form of the startle pattern and that, sadly, in many elderly people this pattern has become a fixed way of being.

Fortunately, we do have a choice in the matter. The significance of the Primary Control is that it serves as a key to coordinating the organism as a whole. If we can develop an understanding of the subtleties of balancing our heads, we can then begin to take responsibility for our righting reflexes, thereby freeing ourselves from fixed attitudinal responses. In other words, as we learn consciously to contact our balanced resting state, we increase the possibility that our actions will be fresh responses to the moment rather than predetermined by the unnoticed remnants of our past.

Checkpoints

Why is it so difficult to 'stand up straight' for more than a minute or two?

What types of experiences cause you to enter the startle pattern?

Do you ever use language that expresses an intuitive understanding of the Primary Control? (ie. phrases such as 'a well-balanced person', 'on the level', 'upright', 'straightforward', 'stand up for oneself', 'get your head together'). Can you think of other examples?

Unreliable sensory appreciation

Everyone wants to be right, but no one stops to consider if their idea of right is right.

Except in cases of parapsychic phenomena, it is safe to say that the body is always the locus of perception and that the quality of an individual's perception depends directly on how his body is functioning. It therefore follows that habitual interference with the right working of the Primary Control must have a distorting effect on perception and prevent, to quote Rudolf Magnus again, 'all the senses of the body regaining their precise relation to the outer world'. The root of such interference, however, lies in the disturbance of our precise relation to our inner world, in particular to our kinaesthetic sense. This, the most intimate of all the senses, provides us with information on our weight, position and movement.

Alexander found that habitual misuse adversely affected the reliability of his kinaesthetic sense and that, most startling of all, his feeling of 'rightness in action' was untrustworthy. In other words he could not be sure that he was doing precisely what he thought he was doing. It is unlikely that he would ever have discovered this had he not been trying to learn something new with the help of an objective method of monitoring his progress that required him to act in a way that was contrary to his established habit. Without seeing it in the mirror, he probably would not have believed that he was not doing what he thought he was doing.

At first Alexander thought that he had merely discovered a personal idiosyncracy, but his teaching experience soon made him realize that 'debauched kinaesthesia' was an almost universal problem, and a particularly insidious one, since by its very nature it eludes awareness. Since kinaesthetic information is a determining factor in our perception of Use, it follows that any interference with kinaesthetic functioning will have a distorting effect on our awareness of ourselves. Our bad habits, such as slumping or breathing through the mouth, most of which operate unconsciously, will come to feel familiar and indeed will become indistinguishable from ourselves. Accepting his Nobel Prize, Nikolaas Tinbergen offered a scientific explanation of how bad habits come to feel right:

> There are many strong indications that, at various levels of integration, from single muscle units up to complex behaviour, the correct performance of many movements is continuously checked by the brain. It does this by comparing a feedback report that says 'orders carried out' with the feedback expectation for which, with the initiation of each movement, the brain has been alerted. Only when the expected feedback and the actual feedback match does the brain stop sending out commands for corrective action.
>
> Already the discoverers of this principle... knew that the functioning of this complex mechanism could vary from moment to moment with the internal state of the subject.... But what Alexander has discovered beyond this is that a lifelong misuse... can make the entire system go wrong. As a consequence reports that 'all is correct' are received by the brain when in fact all is very wrong. A person can feel at ease, for example, when slouching in front of a television set, when in fact he is grossly abusing his body.[26]

I have often observed the practical aspects of this problem in both myself and others. Perhaps the most striking example concerns the pupil who comes for lessons with a posture that can only be described as 'crooked'. Say, for instance, he is hunched forwards so that he appears to be leaning. When he is given the experience of a new balanced way of using himself that results in a relatively erect posture his response is almost invariably, 'But I am falling backwards!' (At this stage in the Alexander Technique lessons a mirror can be employed with great effect.)

Another practical example concerns our inaccurate understanding of the amount of muscle tension or energy needed to perform even the simplest of movements. In one of my early lessons in the Technique, my teacher was guiding me through the movement from sitting to standing. I became aware that my idea of how to stand involved a persistent tendency to shorten my neck muscles and push on the floor with my legs and feet. Using his hands, the teacher helped me to prevent the reactions which predisposed me to these unnecessary tension habits. When the time came to stand, however, I felt that standing was simply not possible from my new configuration. My idea of standing was associated with a certain amount of muscle tension. When this muscle tension was not present, standing as I knew it ceased to be a possibility. The teacher suggested that I think of the direction in which I wanted my head to go in space while he continued to aid the prevention of my habitual misuse with his hands. He said, 'I will count to three and on three you will stand.' 'No chance,' I thought. At the count of three I stood, but it was standing as I had never experienced it before. The movement seemed to have done itself.

This demonstrates what Alexander called 'going from the known to the unknown', an idea that provides the key to understanding how we can make fundamental changes in our behaviour. Our feeling of what is kinaesthetically right or appropriate can be shown to be unreliable. This 'debauched kinaesthesia' is the major influence in what Alexander called 'unreliable sensory appreciation'. Other factors which he considered contributed to this condition included unwholesome diet and bad reading habits. As an example of the harmful effects of diet, he cited in particular the widespread custom of giving children sugar, often in excessive quantities, as an inducement to eating. This he believed led to debauched sense of taste. Imagine his opinion on the effects of spending hours every day watching television or

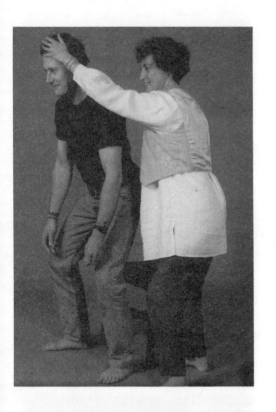

UNRELIABLE SENSORY
APPRECIATION

Even in our most basic actions, such as sitting, bending and standing, we have developed habits which lead us into an inaccurate assessment of the effort needed.

Here the teacher encourages her pupil to keep his length while moving from one position to another. She is giving him a new standard of rightness. He can absorb this directly from the kinaesthetic experience provided by the teacher's hands.

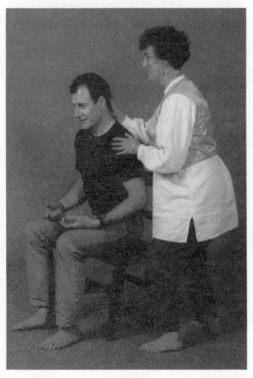

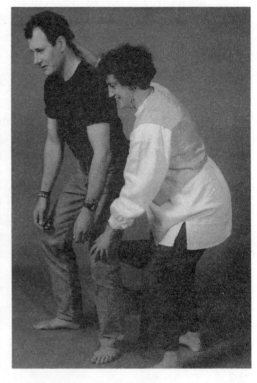

listening to 'heavy-metal' music.

Our sensory mechanisms provide the 'stuff' for our conceptions of ourselves and the world. If the information we receive
from our senses is distorted, then clearly our ideas will be
distorted as well. Dewey recognized the importance of this factor
when he wrote:

> [Alexander's] principle is badly needed, because in all matters
> that concern the individual self and the conduct of its life there
> is a defective and lowered sensory appreciation and judge-
> ment, both of ourselves and our acts, which accompanies our
> wrongly adjusted psychophysical mechanisms... We have
> become so used to it that we take it for granted. It forms, as he
> has clearly shown, our standard of rightness. It influences our
> every observation, interpretation, and judgement. It is the one
> factor which enters into every act and thought.[27]

Alexander continually stressed the importance of accurate sensory
appreciation. One of his teaching aphorisms was that 'feeling,
when it is right, is of much more use than what they call mind'.
As our sensory appreciation improves we may find that we are
getting clearer messages about our true needs. We begin to know
'sensorily' what is right for us. This phenomenon can manifest
itself on a number of different levels, from knowing what it is
right to eat at a particular time to knowing if we have found a
suitable marriage partner.

A striking example of the practical effects of improved sensory
appreciation was provided by a pupil of mine. She was a dancer
recommended to me by a friend of hers who had suggested that
the Technique might help her bad back. When she arrived for
her first lesson, I was immediately struck by the aggressive
demeanour and air of cynicism that accompanied her brusque
physical movements. Yet, in spite of appearances, the session
went well: her back soon felt better, her expression softened, and
she began to experience the classic sensation of lightness and
ease. Her outward toughness was, as I had expected, only a thin
veneer. What I did *not* expect was what occurred thereafter. That
same evening she telephoned me to say that she was feeling

slightly disorientated and was concerned to find herself unable to smoke cigarettes. She simply could not bring herself to do it. I assured her that the effects of the first lesson would wear off and she would soon be able to resume her habit, but she continued with her lessons and of her own accord stopped smoking. Of course, not everyone responds so dramatically, but all of us can begin to question and improve our sensory standard of rightness if we so choose.

My own understanding of 'sensory appreciation' has evolved gradually over a number of years as part of my attempts to understand myself better and get in touch more closely with my feelings and reactions. My path to this goal has often been obstructed by a conflict between the things I have been conditioned to think and feel (that familiar variety of 'oughts' and 'don'ts' imposed by family and society) and my incompletely reasoned responses to them. Observations of friends, pupils and people in general convince me that I am not alone in having this problem. According to one spiritual teacher whose writings I have come across, the path to self-realization involves finding out what one's true needs are and then fulfilling them. Of course the key phrase here is 'true needs'. Discovering one's true needs is no easy trick; all kinds of excess and silliness are indulged in under the guise of 'doing what one really feels like'. If our sensory appreciation is inaccurate we cannot be sure of what our true needs are, but as our standard of rightness develops, intuition begins to be a more valuable tool, and it becomes more difficult to fool ourselves.

Alexander improved the reliability of his 'standard of rightness' by exploring unknown sensory territory, with reason as his guide. Fortunately we have teachers available today to help with this journey from the known into the unknown. To improve our sensory standard we must temporarily suspend the judgements we make on the basis of it and be prepared to experience something beyond habit. This process of suspending judgement is an essential part of the Alexander Technique. It involves the cultivation of an objective and detached awareness that will enable us to apply the experimental method in studying our own behaviour. This takes some courage, as it may lead us to question our basic assumptions, but if we persevere our living and learning can evolve from a process of superimposing one habit on another to one of fundamental change and development.

Checkpoints

Have you ever discovered (perhaps through feedback from a coach or seeing yourself on video) that, like Alexander, you were not doing what you thought you were doing?

How do you know when you are 'too tense'?

How reliable is your intuition? Do you consult it regularly? How can you make your intuition more reliable?

What are your true needs?

Inhibition

The right thing does itself.

In the final chapter of *The Ascent of Man,* Jacob Bronowski wrote, 'We are nature's unique experiment to make the rational intelligence prove itself sounder than the reflex.' Bronowski implied that the success or failure of this experiment depended on the basic human ability to interpose a delay between stimulus and response. He pointed out that, 'In Man, before the brain is an instrument for action it has to be an instrument for preparation.' This ability to stop, to delay our response until we are adequately prepared to make it, is what Alexander calls inhibition.

Alexandrian inhibition is not to be confused with the Freudian concept. Freud's use of the term refers to the suppression of an instinctive desire by the super-ego. Alexander's concept is a matter of common sense – writ large. 'Stop, look and listen' is familiar advice. What Alexander did was to translate this advice into a practical technique based on the natural functioning of the organism. He found that if one refused to respond in an habitual way the Primary Control would function properly, thereby ensuring the best possible balance of mind and body.

This discovery was made when Alexander found that the cause of his voice problem was something he was doing with himself. He was unable to prevent his habitual response by doing something else and had to 'stop off at its source' the psychophysical reaction to the stimulus to recite in order to allow real change to occur. This 'stopping off' process does not involve 'freezing' in place or suppressing spontaneity. Rather, it is a matter of consciously refusing to respond in a stereotyped manner so that true spontaneity can manifest itself. How can the right thing happen if we are still doing the wrong thing? Obviously we have

59

to stop the wrong thing first. This is easy to understand but very difficult to practise.

Alexander pupils often ask for a list of things they can do to improve their Use. It is a while before they understand that the Alexander Technique does not involve doing anything new, at least as we usually understand doing. It is a process of stripping away the things we have imposed on ourselves so that the organism can work naturally and our reason can function without distraction.

Alexander's discovery of the importance of inhibition in human behaviour paralleled a similar discovery in neurology. In *The Integrative Action of the Nervous System*, Sir Charles Sherrington wrote, 'There is no evidence that inhibition of a tissue is ever accompanied by the slightest damage to the tissue; on the contrary, it seems to predispose the tissue to greater functional activity thereafter.'[28] Elsewhere he stated, 'In all cases, inhibition is an integrative element in the consolidation of the animal mechanism to a unity. It and excitation together compose a chord in the harmony of the healthy working organism.'[29] In addition, Frank Jones has written that 'inhibition is the central function of a nervous system which, when it functions well, is able to exclude maladaptive conflict without suppressing spontaneity.'[30]

The primitive vertebrate has a limited range of behaviour and a correspondingly simple nervous system. More complex forms of life demand more sophisticated nervous systems. Inhibition allows higher animals to integrate the numerous stimuli of their environment. This inhibitory mechanism can be observed in the action of a cat stalking its prey. The cat, in Alexander's words, 'inhibits the desire to spring prematurely and controls to a deliberate end its eagerness for the instant gratification of a natural appetite.'[31]

In a cat, as in other animals, inhibition is an instinctive, automatic process. Humanity by contrast has the potential to make this faculty subject to conscious control. Alexander believed that this was necessary if we are to cope with our rapidly changing environment. As our direct dependence on the body to attain subsistence has decreased, our instincts have become increasingly unreliable, and it has become necessary for us to use conscious powers to fill the gap left by their degeneration.

Civilization in the late twentieth century provides continual high-level excitement for the senses. Newspapers, television, video, films, billboards and machinery of all kinds are an almost permanent source of stimulation. Modern communications, especially the telephone, fax and television, extend our senses and open the way to a wider range of assault. The information super-highway threatens to run us over with informational noise. Humanity has more possibilities, more options, than our ancestors can ever have dreamed of. Increased possibilities have brought corresponding changes in the structure of society. Our lives are not as pre-planned as those of our grandparents were. Whereas religious and moral dogma combined with limited material wealth once dictated the course of life, today these limitations have relaxed and we have much more freedom to choose what we will do with our lives. To utilize this freedom constructively we must obviously learn to respond with discrimination to the massive stimulation we receive; we must choose those elements of our environment that are worth responding to.

These choices are important because they affect our functioning. The experience of being 'all wound up' is a common one in our culture; but how do we wind ourselves up? The simple answer is that we stiffen our necks and literally throw ourselves off balance in unconscious response to many aspects of our environment. Our nerves become 'jangled' and our capacity for inner quiet is diminished by the pounding to which we subject our senses. Alexander does not suggest that we should return to more primitive, 'natural' conditions of life but rather that we should take more care about the manner of our reactions. The prevalence of nervous breakdowns and dependence on tranquillizers suggests that we should heed his advice.

Of course we pay lip service to the idea of stopping and thinking before reacting, but this usually takes the form of an admonition or an appeal to the intellect. We do not receive a systematic, practical training in conscious inhibition, and consequently we do not exploit the full potential of our inhibitory powers in preserving our psychophysical balance.

The Alexander Technique develops this inhibitory power in a

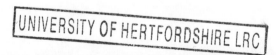

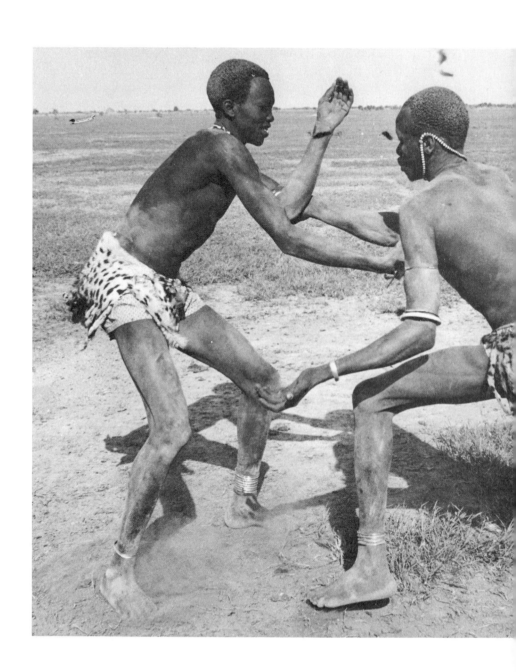

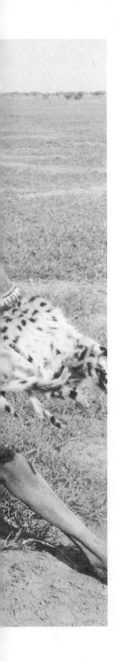

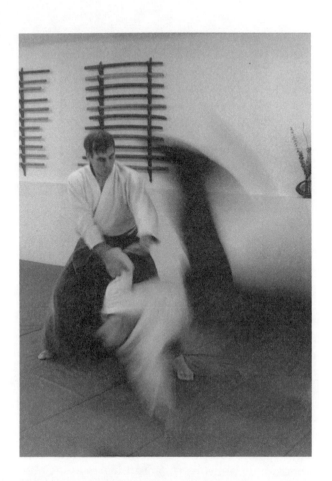

INHIBITION

Martial arts offer a unique context for exploring inhibition. Most people respond to an attack by entering into the 'startle pattern'. The Africans remain free from the tendency to contract and stiffen when exposed to the stress of sparring. Instead, they move with remarkable ease and economy of effort.

The art of aikido requires participants to 'expect nothing, be ready for anything'. This centered freedom-to-respond is predicated on inhibiting the entire neuromuscular habit pattern associated with conflict.

way that involves the whole organism rather than the intellect
alone. The teaching of inhibition often begins when the teacher,
placing her hands in such a way as fully to support one of the
pupil's arms, says something like, 'Please let me take the weight
of your arm: I would like you to let me move the arm without any
help from you at all.' After agreeing, the pupil almost invariably
responds by interfering with the movement, often at a surpris-
ingly gross level. Once this process of interference has been
pointed out, the student can begin to use her powers of attention to prevent the unnecessary response, the teacher providing
feedback about her success.

In the early stages of a course of Alexander lessons, the pupil's
main responsibility is to avoid any unnecessary reaction to the
teacher's hands and to give up her attempt to 'help' the teacher.
In Alexander jargon this is called 'leaving oneself alone'. The
teacher manually guides her pupil into a more balanced Use of
her Primary Control and then takes her through a few simple
movements. She monitors the distribution of tension in the pupil
and helps her to become aware of the ways in which she is interfering with her natural functioning. This is achieved through a
subtle process of tactile feedback and guidance combined with
discussion. The discussion is not a diagnosis; rather, the teacher
uses words in such a way as to enable the pupil to understand for
herself the manifestations of her habitual interference.

As the pupil's experience increases, she can begin to see the
'mental' manifestation of her habitual reactions. She can see, for
instance, how her idea of 'stand up' is associated with a tendency
to tense her neck, and so on. Some teachers play a game with
pupils in which they say something like, 'In a minute, I am going
to ask you to say "hello", but I would like you to do nothing in
response.' When the teacher says, 'Please say "hello",' the pupil
generally responds either by saying 'hello' or 'hell...' or 'h...',
or simply by overtensing her larynx. Eventually the pupil learns
not to respond at all. My own students are often amazed that I
know when they are thinking about standing up or sitting down
or making some other movement. They often ask if the Alexander
Technique gives me the ability to read minds. It doesn't, but the
preparatory tension patterns (postural 'sets', in technical

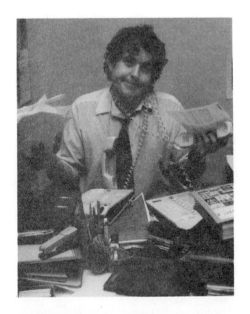

The experience of being 'all wound up' is a common one in our culture; we stiffen our necks and literally throw ourselves off balance in unconscious response to many aspects of our environment. Our nerves become 'jangled' and our capacity for inner quiet is diminished.

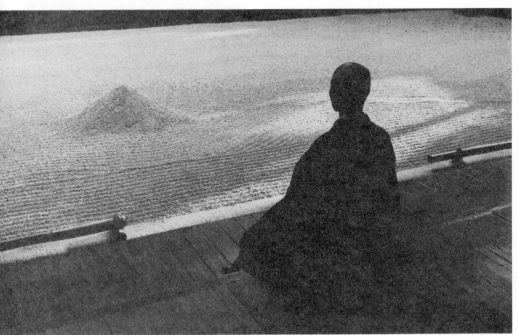

language) that manifest themselves when people are thinking about moving are as clear as daylight. As the student's awareness of these sets increases he refines his ability to say 'no' to his habit.

A pupil develops the ability to stop responding in his habitual way, when he so chooses, first through his own motivation, insight and powers of attention and, second, with the help of manual guidance. The teacher's hands serve not only to prevent interference with the Primary Control but also to convey a quieting, calming influence. In addition, the heightened kinaesthetic experience that often follows improved functioning of the Primary Control helps to develop awareness and coordination. This experience is characterized by a sense of lightness and ease. Habitual tension patterns stand out in a figure-ground relationship against the new kinaesthetic background, making them more accessible to our power to say 'no'.

Alexander believed that inhibition was the foundation of his work:

> Boiled down, it all comes to inhibiting a particular reaction to a given stimulus. But no one will see it that way. They will see it as getting in and out of a chair the right way. It is nothing of the kind. It is that a pupil decides what he will or will not consent to do![32]

Although lessons in the Technique can provide a valuable form of therapy, their real value and purpose comes when they are applied to our daily lives. The extent to which we utilize our Alexander experience is entirely up to us. As Alexander once remarked, 'The teacher will do the best he can for you... but he can't get inside your head and control your reactions for you.'

Perhaps I can make the whole business clearer by giving an example from my own experience. I know that under stress I fall into habitual patterns of reaction. One of the most noticeable manifests itself when I am about to give a lecture or juggling performance: tense neck, raised chest, tightened calf muscles that lift my heels off the ground, sweating hands, faster heart beats, thoughts darting through my mind. I recall one incident in particular, when I was to juggle before four hundred people in the Great Hall at Dartington in Devon. A few hours beforehand I noticed the pattern beginning to creep upon me. In the past I had only been aware of it when it was already in full swing. This time I caught it early, before the adrenalin started to pump. I was able to say 'no' to the whole thing. My mind–body coordination was good enough to enable my decision not to tense my neck, raise my chest and so on to take effect; this in turn indirectly prevented autonomic reactions such as sweating hands and rapid heartbeat. Most interestingly, I found that my calf muscles released so that my feet remained squarely on the ground. My thoughts stayed clear and in focus. Worry about the future was replaced with experience of the present. The performance was a success, and even when at one point I dropped four balls I did not panic. In this incident I experienced something resembling free choice, and I am convinced that inhibition played a central role in making it possible.

Checkpoints

What types of stimuli cause you to respond too quickly?

What happens to your mind and body coordination when you respond too quickly?

Do you ever catch yourself responding habitually but find that you can't seem to change?

Direction

The conscious mind must be quickened.

Alexander realized that he had never consciously thought out how to direct his Use of himself and that he had always depended on what felt right. Having recognized that his feeling was not trustworthy, he found that the key to discovering 'the knowledge of the means whereby trustworthiness could be restored to feeling' lay in subjecting himself to a new experience – the experience of trusting his reason rather than his habit, even if this felt awkward.

His experiments taught him that the best conditions of Use were brought about when he released the tension in his neck, so that his head could go forward and up and his back could lengthen and widen. The problem was that he could not *do* this, he could only let it happen. His attempts to 'put' his head forward and up were based on his habitual feeling of rightness, which is why, at the critical moment, he continually failed to maintain the new Use. He realized that he had to give up any attempt to 'do' anything about securing these conditions, at least as he had always understood the word 'doing'.

He reasoned that the best procedure for his purpose was first to inhibit any immediate response to a stimulus (the example he chose was 'to speak a sentence'). Then he would consciously project a psychophysical pattern that can be described in words as 'allow the neck to be free to let the head go forward and up so that the back may lengthen and widen', taking care to inhibit the translation of these directions into habitual muscular action. The elements of the new pattern were to be projected sequentially and simultaneously – 'all together, one after the other'. In other words, he would continue to give directions for the first part (let

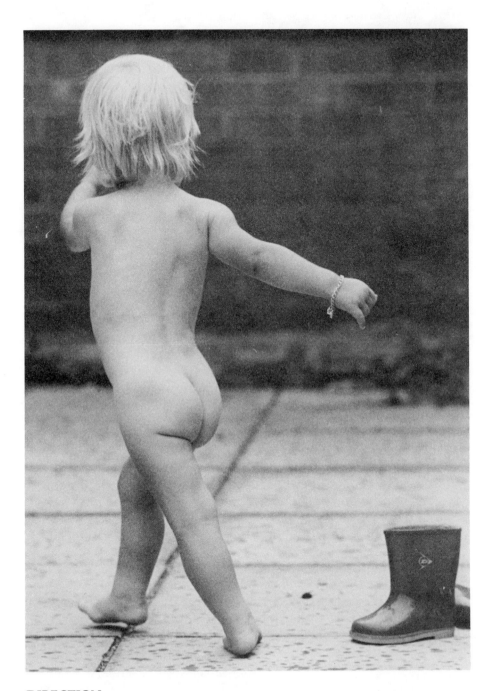

DIRECTION
'Allow the neck to be free to let the head go forward and up so that the back may lengthen and widen.' The expansion which these directions suggest takes place through a sequence of spirals operating throughout the body.

the neck be free) while giving directions for the second part (allow the head to go forward and up), thus building each element into a whole pattern. Projecting conscious directions in this way required a great deal of practice, as indeed was only to be expected, given what Alexander later described as the human race's 'inexperience in projecting conscious directions at all, and particularly conscious directions in sequence'.

The whole business may seem very complex. However, much of an Alexander teacher's training is devoted to simplifying it. The teacher imparts to the pupil an experience of enhanced kinaesthetic perception that helps to raise the pupil's awareness of the manifestations of his own misuse. With such increased awareness, the pupil can learn to inhibit his habitual patterns. In this his teacher's hands not only help to prevent unwanted responses but also remind him of the direction that is wanted. Eventually conscious direction becomes simply a matter of knowing where one is going. Right now, as you read these words, your head, shoulders and knees are all going in some direction. In most cases, the head tends to go back and down in relation to the neck, and the back tends to narrow and collapse. Were you aware of this? Did you choose this pattern of direction? The activity of all your parts reflects the direction of yourself as a whole. An Alexander teacher attempts to help you to organize these parts into a coordinated pattern; when you are working with her, your head *is* going forward and up, your back *is* lengthening and widening. As this experience becomes more familiar, you begin to get a better idea of the directions in which you are going and of where you wish to go.

'Free the neck to let the head go forward and up so the back may lengthen and widen' has wrongly been interpreted as an Alexander mantra, which it most certainly is not. Remembering these words can help to keep one's intention focused, but the experience they represent is clearly beyond words. As a result it is possible to repeat the words constantly without producing any signs of lengthening. Although Alexander's 'directions' may start as a verbal formulation, eventually they become part of one's attitude towards life. This new attitude begins to make sense when we consider that our entire lives take place within a gravitational field that is continually pulling us down. In his book *On Growth and Form*, the biologist D'Arcy Thompson wrote:

> Man's slow decline in stature is a sign of the unequal contest between our bodily powers and the unchanging force of gravity which draws us down when we would fain rise up. We strive against it all our days, in every movement of our limbs, in every beat of our hearts. Gravity makes a difference to a man's height, and no slight one, between the morning and the evening; it leaves its mark in sagging wrinkles, drooping mouth and hanging breasts, it is the indomitable force which defeats us in the end, which lays us on our death bed and lowers us to the grave.[33]

This depressing picture need not be the case. The human organism has a reflex mechanism that effortlessly supports the body against gravity. The Alexander directions set out to 'energize' this mechanism, with which our misuse has interfered. In a word, direction becomes a matter of thinking: 'up'.

Let us consider this 'energizing' quality of thought a little more. Walter Carrington described in a lecture a scene familiar to most Alexander teachers:

> You are taking a pupil and you say, 'I want you to think of your head going forward and up'; that obviously being a direction. You then try and explain to them and show them. After a while they will turn round and say, 'Oh, I see, you only want me to think of it, you don't want me to try and do it.' They say it in such tones as indicate that from their point of view there is a world of difference between doing and thinking... that to do something is practical, tangible, concrete, really down to earth; doing something is what we all understand; but thinking something, this is pretty nebulous, non-effective, vague, all the rest of it. In other words, there is not the same quality of reality between thinking something and doing something.

Carrington made these observations when introducing a discus-

71

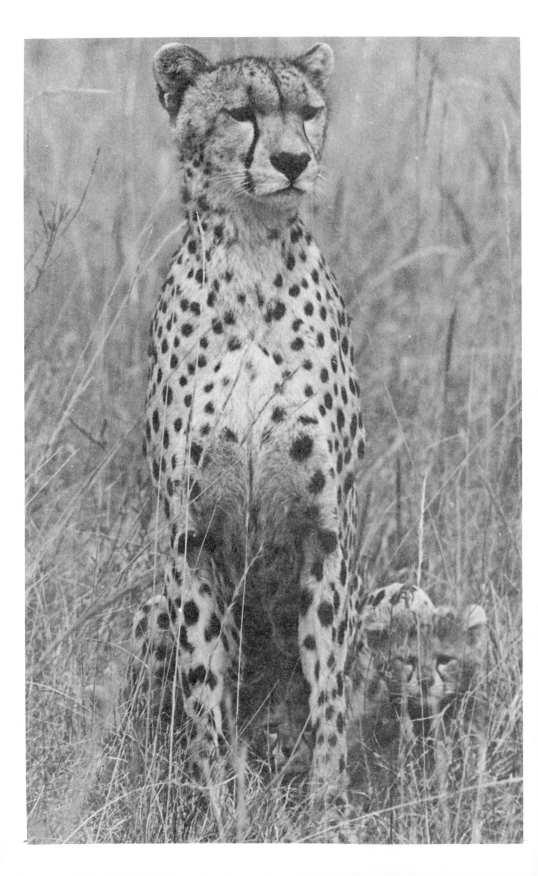

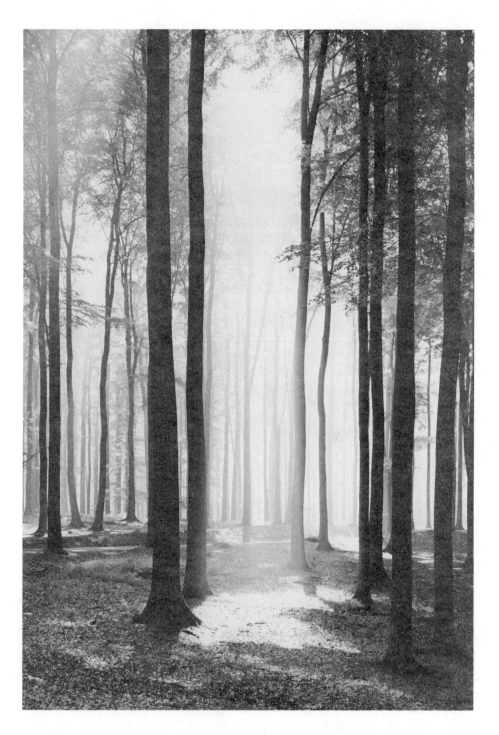

The Alexander Technique encourages a natural, effortless sense of 'up'.

sion of a piece of research presented in an article in *New Scientist* by Professor John Basmajian entitled 'Conscious Control of Single Nerve Cells'. This suggested a much closer relationship between thinking and doing than had been supposed until then. In order to understand Basmajian's work, it is necessary to describe, if only in a simple manner, the way muscles operate.

Every muscle is made up of a vast number of muscle fibres and motor nerves. Each individual nerve cell, or motoneurone, originates in the spinal cord. The axone, or nerve connection, extends from the cord to a bundle of muscle fibres where it splits to make a connection with a part of each fibre called the motor end plate. The nerve cell, axone and fibre bundle (complete with end plates) together comprise a single motor unit. The motor unit is stimulated by an electrical impulse that originates in the brain, travels down the spinal cord along the axone, and results in the contraction of its particular fibre bundle. The action of muscles is the result of the concerted firing of a particular pattern of individual motor units.

Basmajian attached extremely fine electrodes to individual motor units and wired the electrodes to an oscilloscope and an audio-amplifier. In this way he was able to record the electro-contractile pattern of each motor unit. (This process is known as electromyography.) He found that each unit displayed its own characteristic pattern and that this pattern could always be distinguished from that of other units by its shape and by the distribution of 'spikes' on the oscilloscope and the corresponding 'popping' sound recorded on the audio-amplifier. With this information, Basmajian discovered that 'just by thinking about it' the pattern of individual motor units could be changed. The electrical discharge of single motoneurones could be inhibited or increased at will. He reported: 'Most persons became so skilled that they could produce a variety of rhythms such as doublets, triplets, galloping rhythms and even complicated drum roll and drum beats.'[34] A few subjects, including Basmajian himself, were able to recall specific units into activity without the help of the feedback equipment. He added, 'To this day I cannot put into words how I was able to call three different motoneurones unerringly into activity in the total absence of the artificial aids.'

74

Alexander's belief in the 'energizing' power of conscious direction takes on new substance in the context of this research. In his lecture Walter Carrington asked, 'What is the basic difference between choosing to play a rhythm and thinking I'll let my head go forward and up?' We do not really understand how either of these processes works, but, as Carrington added, 'What is clear is that the response you get is a response to wishing, a response to volition.'

To bring the experience of direction on to the conscious level it is almost essential to work with an Alexander teacher, but the reader can obtain a more specific and practical impression of the process by carrying out the following procedure. Direct your attention to your right hand *without moving it at all* in space. Focus on the index finger of the right hand as if you were *intending* to point the finger still further in the direction in which it is already pointing, but remember *not to move it at all*. Look at whatever your finger is pointing towards and sharpen the thought of your finger pointing towards it. This act of attention alone may have produced a change in the muscle tone of the finger. If you keep attending to your *intention* to point your finger while you continue to read you will probably notice that the same subtle yet heightened degree of muscle tone can be maintained. When your attention is drawn away from your finger, the heightened tone decreases, although it is possible to bring it back at will at any given moment. With practice the altered state of tone can be maintained in the background of awareness while continuing to read or to do any other activity. Although this demonstration affects only an isolated part of the musculature, it does help to illustrate the nature of the relationship between attention and muscle tone which is the key to direction.

Attention is very different from what is usually called concentration. Concentration is often associated with a state of over-tension manifested by a furrowed brow and interference with breathing, almost as though one were trying to hold everything in place so as to be able to focus totally on a certain aspect of one's surroundings. Attention in the Alexandrian sense involves a balanced awareness of oneself and one's surroundings with an easy emphasis on whatever is particularly relevant at the moment.

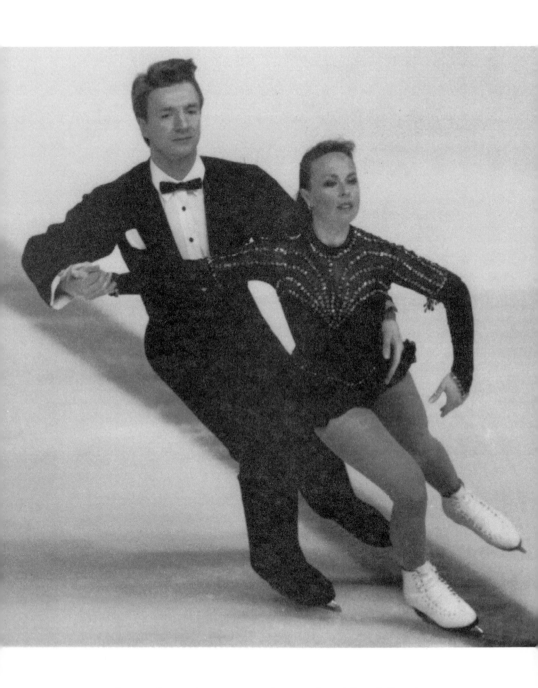

Jayne Torvill and Christopher Dean: perfect synchronicity of direction.

Frank Jones has compared the process with spotlights on a lighted stage: the general surroundings are visible, while different parts receive greater emphasis according to their particular relevance. Alexander found that most people were unable to direct their attention and as a result suffered from 'mind wandering' or over-fixated concentration. Learning to apply the Alexander directions provides an invaluable experience in controlling one's powers of attention. Attention can become something we give rather than something we have to pay.

In order to help students who have difficulty directing their attention, some Alexander teachers employ creative visualization and imagination procedures. A pupil might be asked, for example, to visualize his head floating like a helium balloon or to think of his back smiling. These images are just tools to be used in a specific moment or situation. Creative visualization is not a substitute for direction, but it can be a valuable supplement.

A fascinating study by the psychologist Alan Richardson illustrates the power of the visualization process. Richardson chose three groups of people at random and measured their performance at basketball free-throw shooting. For twenty days, the first group spent twenty minutes a day practising free throws; the second group did not practise at all; the third group did not practise either, but they did spend twenty minutes a day visualizing themselves scoring free throws. At the end of the twenty days, Richardson measured their performance again. The first group had improved by 24 per cent, the second group did not improve at all, and the third group, the visualizers, had improved by 23 per cent. Experiments with dart throwing, figure skating, karate and other activities have shown similar results.

Since every visualization or thought has immediate physiological effects, choosing what one thinks becomes increasingly important. Sorting out what one thinks and wants is an incredibly complex process. The Alexander Technique does not magically clear our thoughts and integrate our desires, but it does focus attention on the importance of the problem while giving us a way of working on it.

• • •

Checkpoints

What is the difference between concentration and attention?

Does your mind wander? What happens to your body when your mind wanders?

Describe the role that gravity plays in your life.

What is the difference between relaxation and collapse?

Ends and
means

*When you've got it, be prepared to throw it
away... throw it away and get it again.*

Alexander's aim was to discover a method of dealing with a
problem of habit and change. He first tried to change his habit
directly by putting his head forward and up because he assumed
that he could do what he thought he was doing. When he found
that he could not, he realized that this assumption was a delusion
and that a fundamental change of habit could only be achieved by
considering the organism as a whole. He knew that the balanced
relationship of his head, neck and torso would organize the rest
of the system and that this balanced relationship could only be
achieved by indirect means. Instead of going directly for his end
(speaking the sentence), Alexander first had to stop and inhibit his
habitual response. In order to ensure that the habitual response
remained inhibited he had to practise the projection of conscious
direction.

In the process of refining this method, Alexander discovered
that it was necessary to 'keep his options open' right through
the critical moment. In other words, he found it necessary to stop
again and consciously reconsider the aim to be achieved. He
could then choose:

(1) not to respond to the stimulus at all
(2) to do something else, such as lifting his arm, or
(3) to go on to fulfil his original aim and speak the sentence.

Whatever course he chose he would *continue to project the directions
for the maintenance of the new Use.* Alexander found that the experience he had gained in maintaining the conditions necessary for

his new Use when exercising one of the first two options also improved his ability to maintain these conditions when he chose the third, or original, option. Continued practice brought him, at last, to the point at which his conscious, reasoning direction was dominating his unreasoning, instinctive direction.

This procedure shows that Alexander always emphasized the *process* of attaining his goal, rather than a narrow focus on the goal itself, an approach which differs from that ordinarily taken in dealing with the material world. We all know that the way to drive a nail into a piece of wood is to hit it directly on the head. The problem starts when we apply this kind of thinking to ourselves, particularly if we are trying to bring about some kind of change. The kind of approach characterized by a dance teacher who pushes down on a pupil's raised shoulder, or a drill sergeant who shouts 'chin in, chest up', is of limited value and will probably produce compensatory maladjustment elsewhere.

Each of us is so complex that we must carefully reason the means we employ to reach any goal. Alexander found that most of us let our immediate goals dominate the field of our attention; he called this 'endgaining' or the 'one brain track' method. If we adopt an 'endgaining' approach to changing our habits, the muscles that habitually perform an act will automatically be activated, so that a stimulus such as the idea 'speak a sentence' will result in a misuse of the organism.

Alexander called the indirect method of change the 'means-whereby' approach, which can be defined as 'awareness of conditions present, a reasoned consideration of their causes, inhibition of habitual responses and consciously guided performance of the indirect series of steps required to gain the end.'[35] Stated simply, Alexander's method is about how to achieve our ends intelligently. Dewey discusses the same issue in *Human Nature and Conduct*:

> Recently a friend remarked to me that there was one super-stition current among even cultivated persons. They suppose that if one is told what to do, if the right end is pointed out to them, all that is required in order to bring about the right act is will or wish on the part of the one who is to act.... He

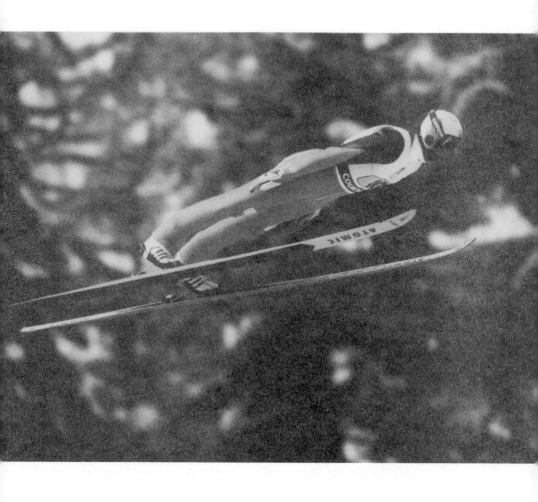

Some activities demand good Use!

pointed out that this belief is on par with primitive magic in its neglect of attention to the means which are involved in reaching an end... We may cite this illustration... A man who has a bad habitual posture tells himself, or is told, to stand up straight. If he is interested and responds, he braces himself, goes through certain movements, and it is assumed that the desired result is substantially attained.... Consider the assumptions which are here made. It is implied that the means or effective conditions of the realization of a purpose exist independently of established habit and even that they may be set in motion in opposition to habit....

A man who does not stand properly forms a habit of standing improperly, a positive, forceful habit. The common implication that his mistake is merely negative, that he is simply failing to do the right thing, and that failure can be made good by an order of will is absurd.... Conditions have been formed for producing a bad result, and the bad result will occur as long as the bad conditions exist.... It is as reasonable to expect a fire to go out when it is ordered to stop burning as to suppose that a man can stand straight in consequence of a *direct* action of thought and desire. Of course something happens when a man acts upon his idea of standing straight. For a little while, he stands differently, but only a different kind of badly. He then takes the unaccustomed feeling which accompanies his unusual stand as evidence that he is now standing right. But there are many ways of standing badly, and he has simply shifted his usual way to a compensatory bad way at some opposite extreme...[36]

Dewey did not fully work out his solution to this problem of 'endgaining' until he studied with Alexander. It was Alexander who gave him the concrete *means* for change which allowed Dewey to conclude:

We must stop even thinking of standing up straight. To think of it is fatal, for it commits us to the operation of an established habit of standing wrong. We must find an act within our power which is disconnected from any thought about standing. We must start to do another thing which on one side inhibits our falling into the customary bad position (inhibition) and on the other side is the beginning of a series of acts which may lead to the correct posture (direction).

Until one takes intermediate acts seriously enough to treat them as ends, one wastes one's time in any effort to change habits. Of the intermediate acts, the most important is the *next* one. The first or earliest means is the most important *end* to discover...

Only as the end is converted into means is it definitely conceived, or intellectually defined, to say nothing of it being executable... Aladdin with his lamp could dispense with translating ends into means, but no one else can do so.[37]

The implications of this approach extend far beyond the issue of standing properly. The Alexander Technique involves a continual emphasis on the means we employ to achieve our aims. The goal of the Technique may be defined as ensuring that our means are always *rationally and physiologically* the best for our purposes. The individual person is the instrument for the realization of his purposes, and the condition of that instrument affects its ability to frame and realize purposes. In seeking to realize our goals, many of us damage and corrupt ourselves. Is it any wonder that our ideals and aspirations often become corrupted in the process?

In an article entitled 'Endgaining and Means-Whereby', Aldous Huxley takes Dewey's discussion a step further:

We have a direct intuition of the value of the highest moral and religious ideals; and we know empirically that the accepted methods of inculcating those ideals are not very effective. Politicians may embark on large scale social reforms designed to improve the world, but these reforms cannot produce more than a fraction of the good results expected of them, unless educators discover means whereby preachers and preached can implement their good intentions and practise what is preached. To build this bridge between idealistic theory and actual practice has proved so difficult that most men and women have hitherto merely evaded the problem.[38]

83

This problem, he adds, is perpetuated by the fact that

> We are all, in Alexander's phrase, 'end-gainers'. We have goals
> towards which we hasten without ever considering the means
> whereby we, as psychophysical organisms, can best achieve
> our purposes... direct attacks cannot in the nature of things be
> effective. True, bad symptoms may be palliated by direct meth-
> ods and a measure of partial good achieved, but these results
> are always attained at a high price. For, if the primary control
> is faulty, all intensive activity, however well intentioned and
> whatever the partial improvements achieved, can only help
> to ingrain habits of improper use. This means that any good
> achieved will be accompanied by harmful by-products, which
> may actually outweigh it, if not immediately, then in the long
> run.

For Huxley the solution lay in the indirect approach. Thus he
concluded:

> In all that concerns life, it is only through the indirect approach
> that the most substantial goods are achieved. Thus religion is
> valueless when it seeks the immediate advantage of the devo-
> tee. To the mystic it is axiomatic that he must first seek the
> kingdom of God and his righteousness.

Huxley's use of the example from religious practice is not acci-
dental, since he believed that the path of the mystic, Christian
or Oriental, was one of the concrete procedures for bridging the
gap between 'idealistic theory and actual practice'. The other
concrete procedure was, in his opinion, Alexander's method.

A brief comparison of the Alexander Technique with a system
of mystical practice may help to make the dynamics of the 'indirect method' clearer. The particular system I have chosen for
comparison is described in Eugen Herrigel's book *Zen in the Art
of Archery*. Herrigel was a German professor who studied under
a Zen Master for six years. His training involved learning archery,
and Herrigel describes how each step in the process of learning to
shoot became an end in itself. The proper way to hold a bow, to

draw the string, to loose the arrow, the proper stance, breathing and, most important, the proper inner state – all these had to be mastered before he was even allowed to think of hitting the target. When it was time to aim at the target, Herrigel was faced with the perplexing task of 'aiming at himself'.

It took years of effort to master the skill. Sometimes Herrigel did hit the target, but he received no approval from the Master. 'Stop thinking about the shot,' the Master would say. 'That way is bound to fail.' 'I can't help it,' Herrigel would reply. The Master explained:

> It is all so simple, you can learn from an ordinary bamboo leaf what ought to happen. It bends lower and lower under the weight of the snow. Suddenly the snow slips to the ground without the leaf having stirred. Stay like that at the point of the highest tension until the shot falls from you. So, indeed, it is: when the tension is fulfilled, the shot *must* fall, it must fall from the archer like snow from a bamboo leaf.[39]

One day Herrigel loosed a shot after which the Master bowed deeply and broke off the lesson saying, 'Just then "It" shot.'

The ultimate aim of Herrigel's quest was to attain the Zen 'everyday mind' described by D.T. Suzuki as 'sleeping when tired, eating when hungry', or, in other words, knowing what one's real needs are. Suzuki has described this state in these words:

> When [it] is attained, man thinks yet he does not think. He thinks like the showers coming down from the sky; he thinks like the waves rolling on the ocean; he thinks like the stars illuminating the nightly heavens; he thinks like the green foliage shooting forth in the relaxing spring breeze. Indeed, he is the showers, the ocean, the stars, the foliage. When a man reaches this age... he is a Zen artist of life. He does not need, like the painter, a canvas, brushes and paints; nor does he require, like the archer, the bow and arrow and target, and other paraphernalia. He has his limbs, body, head, and other parts. His Zen-life expresses itself by means of all these tools

which are important to its manifestation. His hands and feet are the brushes and the whole universe is the canvas on which he depicts his life.[40]

I remember some experiences that have given me a taste of the state that Suzuki describes. One of the easiest to relate happened when I was a member of my college tennis team, before I had ever heard of the Alexander Technique. I was playing in an important match against a difficult opponent. He was leading one set to love, four games to two in the second set. Until then I had been making a gargantuan effort to stay in the match; as the sweat poured down my forehead I thought of my present dilemma and its importance in determining humanity's future evolution, and the humour of the situation occurred to me. Suddenly, my orientation changed from the future (who will win? what will I say if I lose?) to the present (the feel of the racket, the smell of the clay). Without thinking about it, I began to play superb tennis. I won the second set and drew level in the deciding set at six games all. This led to a tie-breaker. I clearly remember my feeling of detachment at the time, despite the fact that my coach and all the spectators had gathered around the court. In the tie-breaker I played the best tennis of my life, winning all the points effortlessly. 'It' won the match.

At 'peak' or 'creative' moments such as this, I find that the distinction between ends and means disappears... I am left with a feeling of the Eternal Present Moment. In the past these experiences came rarely and without conscious intention on my part. Through my involvement with the Alexander Work I have found a systematic, Western method for opening myself to this process of 'non-doing'. My actions are tending more and more to 'slip like snow from a bamboo leaf'.

Just as there are laws of physics that govern the behaviour of objects, so I believe that there are laws of human reaction that can be applied to unlock our highest potential. Alexander discovered some of these laws through the application of the experimental method to his own behaviour. He did it entirely on his own, without reading books on self-knowledge or studying Zen.

● ● ●

Checkpoints

In what aspects of life do you tend to 'endgain'?

How would you apply the archery master's advice, to 'aim at oneself'?

What are the similarities between Alexander's insights and Zen or Taoist thought? What are the differences?

These seven operational ideas:

Use and functioning
The whole person
Primary Control
Unreliable sensory appreciation
Inhibition
Direction
Ends and means

provide a framework for understanding and appreciating Alexander's discovery. The beauty of Alexander's work is more than a set of principles, however profound. He also developed a unique, practical method for guiding pupils to embody these ideas in daily life.

3

Learning
How to
Learn

The essence of the Alexander technique is to make ourselves more susceptible to grace.

F.M. ALEXANDER

Utilizing potential

The physical, mental, and spiritual potentialities of the human being are greater than we have ever realized...

When observing the behaviour of infants, one is struck by the wholeheartedness with which they explore their environment – legs kicking, arms reaching out to the unknown. They seem like little scientists trying to make sense of the world around them. Their mistakes become part of experience, and they are totally undaunted by failure, feeling no disgrace or embarrassment, only a renewed desire to go on exploring.

John Holt, a teacher and the author of *How Children Fail*, has written of his observations of babies and infants:

> They show a style of life and a desire and ability to learn that in an older person we might well call genius. Hardly an adult in a thousand, or ten thousand, could in any three years of his life learn as much, grow as much in his understanding of the world around him, as every infant learns and grows in his first three years.[41]

The quality of an infant's movement and the integrity of its body reflect this attitude. Although their heads are disproportionately large in relation to their bodies and coordination is not fully developed, infants move freely and without undue tension. They sit upright, bend at the knees and lengthen their spines naturally. Placing a hand on a baby's back, one can sense the wholeness of its body, the energy streaming through it.

What happens to this love of learning and psychophysical integrity as the child grows older? Holt answers in this way:

> It is destroyed, and more than by any other one thing, by the process that we misname education – a process that goes on in most homes and schools. We adults destroy most of the intellectual and creative capacity of children by the things we do or make them do. We destroy this capacity above all by making them afraid, afraid of not doing what other people want, or not pleasing, of making mistakes, of failing, of being wrong. Thus, we make them afraid to gamble, afraid to experiment, afraid to try the difficult and unknown.[42]

My own experiences of learning and teaching in both Great Britain and the USA have convinced me of the truth of what Holt says. I attended a middle-class, all white, 'model' elementary school. My high school was inter-racial, urban and 'tough'. College was sophisticated, private and 'progressive'. All were based, in their own way, on fear. Each institution, with varying degrees of subtlety, was a battleground for winners and losers. Until my first year of high school, I tended to be on the losing side and was labelled an under-achiever. I was unhappy and struggled against my teachers; the work seemed boring and meaningless. Gradually I came to realize that with a little bit of effort I could tell my teachers what they wanted to hear. This made life much easier and I became one of the 'winners', in as much as I graduated from high school with honours and was captain of the athletic team and so on.

At university I met others who had reacted in the same way to their high school experiences. The spirit of the time was one of questioning; there was tremendous opposition to the Vietnam War and not only educational but also social, political and religious values were being challenged. I knew that something was not right in society and started to explore possibilities for change. I took part in demonstrations, teach-ins and other forms of protest, but none of these seemed to reach the root of the problem. It became apparent to me that most people, conservative or liberal, were acting out their conditioning, either directly or by reaction. As a result I realized that I had better sort myself out before teaching or preaching, and I changed my course from political science to psychology, hoping to find the key to freeing myself from the dominance of conditioning and habit. However, I was quickly disillusioned by the sterility of rat-chasing behaviourism and conceptual callisthenics. I went on to study philosophy, aiming to get to the bottom of things that way, but instead I got more theory without experience. Realizing the limitations of academic study, I then began to seek guidance from sources based on experience. I discovered the work of Carl Jung, whose life appeared to be a reflection of the things he taught. The picture of human potential revealed in his writings inspired me and I began to experiment with a variety of Eastern and Western techniques for self-development. Eventually I found my way to the International Academy for Continuous Education in the west of England where as part of a self-sufficient community I spent a year learning to apply these techniques to practical, everyday situations. It was at the I.A.C.E. that I was introduced to the Alexander Technique, which was the most concrete method for developing self-observation and self-knowledge I had yet experienced. Having decided to become an Alexander teacher, I found during my training that I began to get a clear idea of the habit patterns that had interfered with my ability to learn. As I began to uncover these patterns I traced their origins back through my university and school days.

I now understand that in achieving external 'success' I had lost touch with the real meaning of learning. I professed to believe in progressive education, but my behaviour, particularly when challenged to learn something new, was anything but progressive and was characterized by rampant endgaining and fear. I generally avoided the new and unfamiliar, concentrating instead on things at which I was already good. Although I was interested in the so-called 'creative' activities such as art and music, I never seemed to have much natural talent and shied away from experimenting with them. I chose not to face my fear of not being good and went instead to concerts and art galleries where I could demonstrate my verbal skills in critical analysis, thus exaggerating my one-sidedness and sacrificing wholeness.

Learning had developed unpleasant associations. I saw it as something difficult, requiring drudgery, persistence and a teacher or school. Worst of all, it was something to be done for reward or external approval, not something that came from myself, for myself. Eventually I realized that all this applied to the way I had tried to learn about self-development.

Although I did benefit from studying other methods, the Alexander Technique was of fundamental importance in my quest to overcome the dominance of habit and to relearn how to learn. This is because the Alexander lesson is essentially an exercise in how to learn. The Alexander pupil has the undivided attention of his teacher, who listens and communicates, not just verbally but with his hands as well. He is learning at least as much as his pupil. Each lesson becomes a living experiment in bringing intelligence into the activities of everyday life. Lessons take place in an atmosphere free from comparison or competition; there are no diagnoses or tests, no black belts or gold stars. The unique feature of a lesson is that the teacher actually gives the pupil the experience of balanced coordination. Like other teaching methods, the Technique involves instruction, demonstration, practice; but I have never discovered any other method in which the desired result is virtually brought about for the pupil. The kinaesthetic experience is a gift, but this gift takes time to understand, and of course the pupil must practise conscious inhibition and direction if he is to make the gift truly his own. Nevertheless, some improvement in coordination is almost inevitable unless the pupil actively resists it.

This experience gives a direct taste of the potential for freedom and grace that lies locked inside us. It can be upsetting to realize that we have so much that has not been used; yet I have had pupils in their sixties and seventies who have begun to change the habits of a lifetime. It is as though poise is there beneath the surface, waiting to be discovered.

Another special aspect of the Technique is that in order to aid this process of discovery the Alexander teacher *must* practise what she preaches. People are all too familiar with crazy psychologists, unhealthy doctors and materialistic gurus. In order to teach the Technique properly, a teacher must work on herself continually. The first two years of her training are devoted almost exclusively to improving her own Use, for only after a certain standard has been reached can work on others begin. Every time a teacher puts a hand on a pupil she must be working on herself, inhibiting her habitual reactions and consciously directing her Use.

The best teachers I have ever had, whatever the discipline, have almost always been people who teach from their own experience. This has been the case with all my Alexander teachers. In order to teach the Technique one must experience the process of change and growth for oneself. There is no other way.

The Alexander lesson takes place on the level of the self. It does not involve learning how to use any equipment except one's own. Learning how to use oneself is basic and immediate, and I have found that it provides a superb model for learning anything.

There are some ways in which I have found the Alexander Technique useful in helping me to utilize my potential to learn:

Dealing with fear

Fear is the biggest block to learning in an integral way. It interferes, both psychologically and physiologically, with an individual's ability to respond freely and to function naturally, abilities essential to integral learning. Fear has long been deliberately used as a teaching device in the armed services and in sports coaching. It gets results, but the long-term effects are always crippling.

We all have our fears: fear of the dark, of failing, of looking silly. Many of them go very deep; they may be rational or irrational, but the insidious thing about them is that they usually function subconsciously. The Technique has helped me to increase my awareness of stereotyped responses to fear. It has given me the means to make my fears more accessible to consciousness. This is the first step in understanding and resolving them and in stopping them from stifling the ability to learn.

Developing attention

The procedure Alexander devised to solve his original problem involved stretching his attention to the limit. As a result of practising this procedure, my ability to give attention freely and easily has increased.

The field of attention is always reflected in the state of one's muscle tone and balance. The improved awareness of these factors that I have achieved through the Technique has increased my ability to monitor my attention and my performance in any activity. Having learnt to 'listen' to myself in this way, I find it has become easier to listen to others, an ability that is usually a great help in learning anything.

Attention to process

There is no way of forcing results in the Technique. Attention must be paid to the means-whereby at every stage. The Primary Control simply cannot be made to work directly.

In most other areas of life endgaining will produce apparent results – which is why we all do it. The problem is that these immediate results are often obtained by sacrificing poise, and this sacrifice takes its toll in the course of time.

I have learnt to pay more attention to the 'how' of things and to include my own poise as a fundamental aspect of my approach to learning.

Going from the known to the unknown

Alexander once said:

> You want to feel out whether you are right or not. I am giving you a conception to eradicate that. I don't want you to care a damn if you're right or not. Directly you don't care if you are right or not, the impeding obstacle is gone.[43]

Alexander found that when pupils were learning to direct themselves they exhibited an almost irresistible urge to 'feel out' the effects of the directions in order to see if they were 'right'. However, faulty kinaesthetic perception makes such efforts futile and they interfere with the efficacy of the directions. In most people the idea 'Am I right?' seems to be associated with a fixed pattern of tension that prevents them experiencing a new and freer balance. In a concrete way, the Technique teaches a pupil to trust reason at the risk of feeling disorientated, to venture from the 'known to the unknown'. This journey necessitates a willingness both to make mistakes and to profit by them that is the essence of learning.

Experimental thinking

When Dewey spoke of 'making the method of intelligence exemplified in science supreme in education' his concern was not so much with the technical aspects of science as with its qualities of impartiality, honesty, freedom, open-endedness, practicality. He believed that the application of the scientific method begins with an individual's confrontation with a real and meaningful problem. I certainly had one of my first real tastes of this method when I learnt to experiment with my own Use, checking my progress by observing myself in the mirror and noting the quality of my breathing.

The Alexander Technique involves a continual attempt to discover and free ourselves from deeper and deeper layers of interference with natural functioning. This never-ending experimental process is guided by the basic principles of the Technique, which are tested in action.

Improved kinaesthesia and coordination

The development of the kinaesthetic reliability and coordination fostered by the Technique makes learning any skill easier from the start. Again, since studying the Technique I have found it much easier to get an accurate conception and 'feel' of a new task. In addition, I find that my body is much more willing and able to follow the instructions it is given.

Non-interference

I was brought up to believe that the harder I tried, the more I would learn. In my Alexander lessons this strategy simply did not work. I could not *do* anything to improve my balance; I had to learn about non-doing. At first this was baffling, but I went on to discover that the solution to many seemingly difficult tasks is not to 'try harder' but to leave oneself alone. The key to learning something new is often in preventing unwanted responses, which

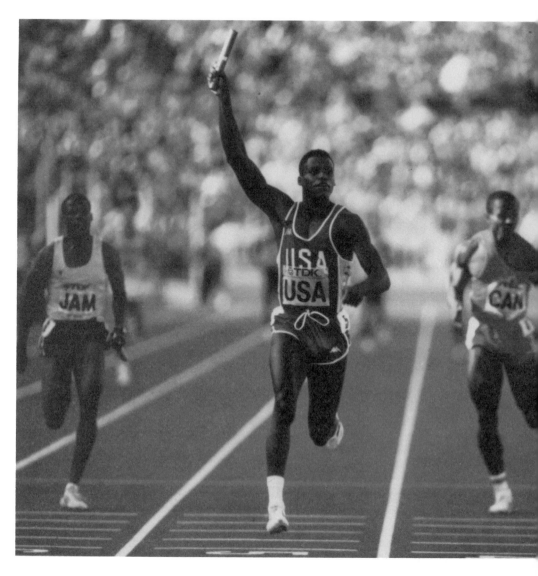

A person's attitude to competition is visible in his face and body. If he responds by narrowing his field of attention, trying hard, and losing his awareness of the present in the struggle to win, he will have tight lips and furrowed brows and his movements will be twisted and jerky. The competitor who, on the other hand, is able to open his attention and not get in his own way will show in his face an openness, alertness and ease, and in his body good alignment, flow and unified power.

And, like Carl Lewis, he will probably win.

leads to the discovery of appropriate effort. My organism now appears to be capable of much more than I had ever imagined it could be – so long as I do not get in the way.

Many of Alexander's discoveries are things that all good teachers know. One writer, reviewing *Man's Supreme Inheritance*, called the Technique 'systematized common sense'. To that definition I would add that it is systematized common sense based on an understanding of the natural functioning of the human being. John Dewey pointed out that the Technique 'bears the same relation to education that education itself bears to all other human activities'. One of my colleagues calls the Alexander work a 'pre-technique', because learning good Use is fundamental to everything else. Like music, the Technique only lives when it is played. It is meant to be applied to life. I have found it useful in helping me do whatever I want as well as I can, as the following examples show.

Learning to sing

One word describes my reaction to being told that singing lessons were to be included as part of the Alexander training course – fear. I had always been told that I wasn't 'musical' and had been led to believe that I was tone-deaf. At Christmas, when the time came to sing carols, I was usually sent off to stir the egg nog. My first meeting with the singing teacher was a disaster for me. Eight of us sat in a circle and were asked, in turn, to sing 'anything'. When my turn came, I refused; I was scared stiff.

When private lessons began the pressure decreased. My teacher was very positive, insisting that I could sing and ignoring my protestations. At first this put me off, but soon I began to see that she was right.

I learnt that if I didn't think too much about pitch, if I didn't try so hard to be 'right', I could begin to hit the correct notes. I observed that my habitual reaction to the ideas 'sing' and 'hit the note' involved a modified form of the startle pattern. (It is not easy to sing with an unduly depressed larynx.) I saw that I was in a vicious circle: my habitual response would interfere with my voice, when I heard the resulting sound I would tense up further, and so on. Obviously I had to stop this at its source. I had to inhibit my habitual response and put my attention on the means-whereby, the process.

My teacher suggested that I drop my jaw, brighten my face and direct my voice to a point across the room. I put my attention on these specific things while keeping the general directions for the best Use of myself in the background of awareness. (This process of juggling attention in action is what Dewey called 'thinking in activity'.) My coordination was good enough to ensure that whenever I remembered a direction it would happen (my teacher informed me that this is not usually the case with pupils who have not had Alexander lessons). At first, however, this was only true when I was dealing with very simple phrases. When I tried to sing high notes or difficult pieces my unreasoned, instinctive direction dominated my intentions. With continued practice I found I was able to maintain the necessary conditions in progressively more difficult phrases. All this work involved new experiences. I had to be prepared to open my mouth and let unfamiliar sounds come out – and this was the hardest of all.

When I managed to avoid my habitual interference and venture into the unknown, the various directions I was giving would merge into an integrated experience. I couldn't believe some of the sounds that were emanating from me.

I now hardly ever miss a note when singing accompanied, my voice quality is improving and I am beginning to find my true voice.

Learning to juggle

I learnt to juggle the hard way. I was given a demonstration, told how to throw the balls up, and left to get on with it. Fortunately, I really wanted to learn. I struggled to keep the balls going, grabbing after them and contorting my body in the process. Nevertheless, it was great fun, and I persisted. After a few months of practising for ten minutes a day I could keep three balls going and do a few tricks. Just as I was beginning to experiment I met a superb juggler who was also a patient teacher. He taught me many technical tricks and provided an excellent model. After a year and a half of intermittent practice, I could do a reasonable routine with three and four balls and was working on five.

At about this time I began to train as an Alexander teacher. It wasn't long before I realized that when juggling I was using about ten times more energy than necessary. Of course, I was already aware that continued practice made the whole process easier; I could certainly manage three balls with much less effort than a year before. However, how the necessary effort had been reduced was a mystery.

The mystery began to clear as I became aware of what I was doing with myself in order to juggle. I observed that I supported myself by leaning on a stiffened left leg and that I overtensed my neck, arms and shoulders while restricting my breathing, particularly during difficult manoeuvres. In particular, I was struck by the amount of tension I created every time I caught a ball. These habits were obviously limiting my progress, and I was beginning to feel that certain tricks were beyond me. Maybe I had reached the limit of my potential. Bad habits were not only interfering with my general functioning, but were also blocking my progress.

In order to experiment with my Use and to give my work on the Technique time to sink in, I stopped practising regularly for a few months. As soon as I started again, I noticed a subtle reduction in the amount of effort required. Perhaps I was only using about seven times more than I needed. When I tried to learn new variations, I was able to get a better 'feel' of what they might be like. Although my habit patterns were still present, their influence had diminished slightly. I became aware that I had always focused my attention on catching the balls rather than on throwing them. This helped to explain why I tensed up while catching.

I now began to see the whole problem in the context of the juggler's ever-present fear of dropping the balls. I had always tried to 'get it right' by going directly for my end: catching the balls. Now I paid more attention to the process, to the throw, inhibiting any attempt to reach for the ball if it didn't land right in my hand, and soon I was juggling with my eyes closed.

The acid test was, of course, public performance. More often than not I would revert to my old habits; but the quality of my juggling had nonetheless definitely improved and my attitude to my fear of dropping the balls was changing. The feeling of panic that used to follow a drop could be controlled by a decision not to respond in a habitual way. Instead of rushing after the ball I would just stand there with a bemused look on my face. Usually the ball would bounce up and I could incorporate it into the rhythm of the act. There was always a member of the audience who said, 'He did that on purpose!' My ability to monitor my performance was also increasing. Not only was I more in touch with my juggling, but I was more aware of the crowd's reaction, my facial expression (grimaces and juggling just don't mix) and my own inner state. I seemed to be more 'centred'. This proved useful when I worked five nights a week as a 'court jester' in a restaurant specializing in 'medieval banquets'. The place was a juggler's nightmare: low ceilings, poor lighting, five hundred drunken tourists, and a bevy of harried 'wenches' and other performers with defective spatial awareness.

Continued work with the Technique has helped to bring me to a point at which I can claim that I only use twice as much energy as I need. Juggling has become as natural as walking. I am currently working on seven balls and on a few tricks that I could never have imagined doing before. None of this would have happened without practice, high motivation and good teachers. My work with the Technique simply provided a systematic method for getting more out of my practice and improving my coordination.

Teaching juggling

The problem of learning to juggle can be solved in a much easier way than the one I originally employed. Because juggling involves a journey into the unknown, Alexander's principles provide a useful guide. I base my juggling classes on the application of inhibition, direction and attention to the means-whereby. A typical first lesson begins with a demonstration and warm-up session. I then give each pupil a ball and ask him to play with it and at the same time to direct his attention to the feel of the ball and the amount of energy he uses to throw it. I then have him throw the ball in various trajectories and observe the effect on his balance, and, most important, I encourage him to get used to dropping the ball and enjoying it.

With this help the students eventually realize that control and balance can best be obtained by keeping the balls within an imaginary box. I then demonstrate the best trajectory for throwing a ball from one hand to the other within the box and ask them to close their eyes and visualize themselves throwing the ball from hand to hand. When they begin to practise, I ask them to avoid reaching for the ball if it is thrown outside the box, as this allows them to retain their balance.

The next stage involves throwing one ball from right to left and one from left to right, symmetrically, in staggered timing. I divide the class into pairs and ask them to practise for a few minutes. The pupil who is not juggling is asked to observe, for his own benefit, the manifestations of his partner's Use (what happens to the head–neck relationship, the breathing and so on). He is also responsible for picking up the balls when they drop. The juggler begins by tossing the balls up in sequence and letting them drop. After some practice, he experiments with catching the first ball while letting the second drop and then with catching the second while the first drops. His responsibility is to attend to the quality of his throw and to inhibit his habitual response to the dropping of the balls, which almost invariably involves lunging after them. If a pupil does this repeatedly he sacrifices whatever equilibrium he has and begins to juggle, 'set' to lunge. When a pupil learns inhibition he starts to see that it is necessary to pause between every few throws in order to find his equilibrium. While the juggler waits for his partner to retrieve the balls he is asked to remember his visualization of what he wants to happen.

One of the biggest obstacles to learning two-ball juggling is the psychophysical preconception that people have of it. The majority of pupils, despite clear demonstrations to the contrary, tend to hand the ball from the left hand to the right instead of throwing it. When they are made aware of this response they are often amazed to find that they weren't doing what they thought they were doing. The pupil can get over this obstacle by pausing between throws and directing his attention to preventing the unwanted response while visualizing what is required.

After an hour or so most people are juggling two balls. At this stage I ask the pupil to put his hands into the ready position for juggling. Then I gently take hold of his wrists and ask him to let me have the weight of his arms so that I can control their movement. I guide his hands through the motion required for three balls, emphasizing the rhythm. I then tell the pupil, 'When I count to three I want you to take the weight of your hands from me, but I want you to do so with as little effort as possible. The way to do this is to leave open the possibility that your hands will fall when I let go.' If the pupil makes any unnecessary tensional adjustments before I reach 'three' I ask him to note it and we start over again. The pupil is exploring unknown sensory territory. Eventually he realizes that he can hold his arms up and throw a ball with much less energy than he had thought.

I finish the lesson by asking everyone to throw three balls in the proper sequence, letting them all drop.

Throughout the session I ask the pupils to direct their attention to their Use of themselves, in particular to observe the effects of their actions on their breathing. I emphasize that once the technical details have been learnt, juggling becomes a matter of avoiding interference with natural functioning.

Pupils often report, 'I was throwing up two balls and all of a sudden the right rhythm "just happened".' After juggling three balls for the first time a sixty-year-old lady once said, 'I've just done the impossible.'

The biggest problem to overcome in teaching juggling is pupils' fear of unfamiliar territory. Most of my students start with the idea that they can't learn; they may think they are too uncoordinated or too old. Those few who have a more positive outlook tend to try so hard that they don't really give themselves a chance. All of them want to 'get it right' from the very beginning. Except for a few extraordinary individuals this is simply not possible. Balls have to be dropped in order to learn. But most people are afraid of dropping the balls; they think it makes them look silly. It does, but they look even sillier when they struggle to catch them before they are ready. Attention to the means-whereby seems to short-circuit these fears, and it also gets results. Working on these principles I have found that almost everyone who stays the course has a good time, learns how to juggle, and also learns something about how to learn anything.

Learning to ride the unicycle

The unicycle is guaranteed to stimulate anyone's fear of falling. The rider is raised off the ground in a precarious balance; he can fall in three hundred and sixty directions! In order to ride properly, the cyclist must keep his bottom firmly on the seat, his upper body erect and his eyes looking forward. Unicycle riding requires an individual to go 'forward and up'; it seems to compel the antigravity mechanism into action. The irony of learning to ride is that fear of falling results in the head being pulled back, which disturbs balance and inevitably causes a fall.

When I first tried to get on a unicycle I fell off immediately. I soon discovered that I could stay up by supporting myself on a wall and, later, by using a broomstick as a cane. But when I tried to ride unsupported, my fear of falling quickly asserted itself. My inhibitory powers could not cope with the overwhelming force of instinct, and I realized that I would have to overcome my fear in order to learn.

I set about doing this by giving up any idea of trying to stay up and instead practised falling off and enjoying it, believing that if I didn't tense up I wouldn't get hurt. When I felt confident that I could fall safely, I started thinking about staying up again, realizing that I had 'nothing to fear but fear itself'. Soon I was able to ride short distances. However, I noticed that whenever my balance became particularly precarious I tended to pull my head back and also lift myself off the seat and put undue pressure on my legs.

Practice with falling made it possible to allow my inhibitory powers to work. By inhibiting my habitual response and directing my bottom down and my head forward and up, I was able to gain control over the unicycle. When this process of 'thinking in activity' is maintained, the unicycle comes to feel like an extension of the spine, the legs being replaced by a wheel.

Learning to speed read

I studied speed reading as part of a week's intensive course in study skills. My original reading speed was 320 words per minute, slightly above the class average.

We began with conditioning exercises, in which pages had to be scanned first one line at a time, then one line forwards one line backwards, two lines at a time, and so on. The progressive increases in speed were paced by a metronome. We were asked to forget about comprehension for the time being and to concentrate on speed, since, if new and faster reading patterns are practised regularly, the brain will eventually learn to decode them. (Anyone can test this idea by holding a book upside down and attempting to read; with a little practice it becomes possible.) Our teacher urged us to practise and to be patient, assuring us that we would eventually be able to comprehend at high speeds, an idea that the majority of the class resisted. Almost everyone seemed to agree that reading without comprehension felt strange; it produced a sense of insecurity that led to a desire to grasp individual words instead of allowing the eyes to scan one or two lines at a time. A number of people became quite upset – and I doubt they would have tried any further if they hadn't paid a substantial fee for the course! I too experienced this desire to grasp at words; it was a powerful habit, and reading in the old way felt much more comfortable. However, I *knew* from my Alexander experience that learning involved a venture into the unknown and I almost welcomed the process.

I continued for three days without much comprehension at all. On the fourth day, I began to understand a little and by the end of the week I was reading 1800 words per minute with good comprehension. Everyone in the class, with one notable exception, experienced a similar improvement. One difference between my classmates and myself was that I didn't suffer as much anxiety in the process.

The one 'notable exception' provides an example of the stultifying effects of preconceived ideas fixed by habit. Ironically, this man was employed as a study skills teacher. He possessed a great deal of theoretical knowledge about learning and spent the entire week arguing against the theories that were behind our teacher's methods. His attitude appeared to be reflected in his body, which was so tense and fixed that it almost hurt to look at him. I guess that all the theory in the world would not have convinced him to have a try, to take a chance. This very bright person had somehow had his ability to learn crippled.

Learning to write

Throughout my career at school and college I found writing (essays, term papers and so on) an excruciatingly painful process. This was largely because the subjects I was usually asked to write about bore little relation to my experience or interests. Even when this was not the case, however, I still found it difficult. I couldn't tolerate the ambiguity that writing necessitates – I felt I needed to see a complete picture of what I would write before I put pen to paper. If I managed to start a paper, I would panic the minute I came up against a problem, throwing my pen down and looking for answers outside myself. Almost everything I wrote in college was produced by joining paraphrased quotes with 'and's. Occasionally I would get my ideas in, but usually I was under too much pressure really to be able to think about what I wrote.

Ironically, this book, which is about learning, represents the first real learning experience I have had in the context of writing. I started it with a good deal of apprehension. Soon I realized that I couldn't write about these principles without applying them to writing. If I was to have any integrity in the matter, I had to attend to the means-whereby.

Whenever a feeling of panic has arisen (which it often has) I have stopped and directed my attention to not interfering with the Primary Control. Usually when I return to writing, the problem no longer seems as serious. I have become much more willing to write without feeling sure that I am seeing the whole picture. I find that by simply writing down whatever comes into my head one idea leads naturally to the next and the whole creates itself. I am still free to throw things out and have begun to see that if I do not get too tense the words begin to flow. I find myself getting truly interested in what I am writing.

The experience of writing in this way has enabled me to confront many of my ideas and preconceptions. It has increased my understanding of my work and has opened up whole new areas for myself. It hasn't been easy, and occasionally the pressure has got on top of me; but on the whole, it has been an exhilarating journey into the unknown.

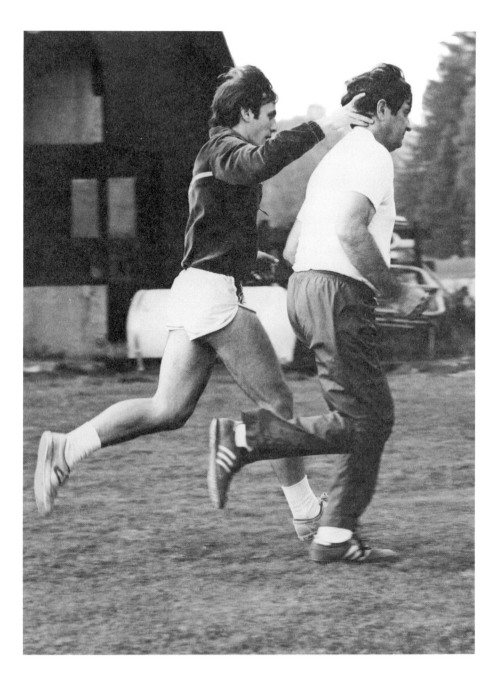

The author's hand is elastic and alive, and able to convey the desired stimulus because the way he is using himself is light, free and expanding. This stimulus transforms the pupil's experience of running from being a heavy, contracting, downward pulling activity to becoming a light, upwardly expanding, free flow of movement.

Learning to run

I have never been particularly enthusiastic about running. It was a tortuous but essential part of training for the different sports I played at school, but I never understood how people could actually enjoy it. This attitude has in no way been changed by the hordes of purple-faced, pulled-down joggers who have invaded our streets and parks in recent years.

Nevertheless, having witnessed the elegance and beauty of Linford Christie, Carl Lewis, Florence Griffith-Joyner and other great runners, I felt that running could be more than a way of working up a sweat and developing the ability to cope with pain.

I was very fortunate, therefore, that Paul Collins was one of my Alexander teachers. Collins represented Canada in the Commonweath Games Marathon in 1950 and in the Olympics in 1952. In 1979, on his fifty-third birthday, he ran 53 miles. Since then he has set 12 world records for distance running in his age group. Paul organized weekly running sessions for his private Alexander pupils, training-course students and friends. Working with him completely changed my attitude towards running, as well as my style. Indeed, it was through this work that I learnt that there was such a thing as a 'style' of running.

My old style was like that of the typical athlete: torso leaning forward, head thrown back, shoulders rolling and legs overworking. All good runners and coaches know that the upright posture is most efficient. Not only did Collins tell me this, he actually 'gave' me the experience. He started by working with me while I was standing still, helping to activate my anti-gravity reflexes. As I started to go 'up' he would launch me into running and then run alongside me with his hand lightly on my neck, helping to prevent interference with the Primary Control. The result was almost incredible. I ran in a completely new way, floating along effortlessly. My legs had much less to do in order to keep me going – they seemed to disappear. My awareness of the environment passing by as I ran was heightened. Freed to a great extent from the drag on my body, I found more energy to appreciate the flow of the ground and trees as I ran along. Suddenly I understood the joy of running. When I run on my own now the results aren't always as dramatic as this initial experience, but I do experience running as a lighter, easier process – and not just on the physical level.

I have profited greatly from my study of the Alexander Technique. It has been instrumental in helping me to relearn how to learn. But it is not a panacea or a magic carpet. Although the principles of the Technique are simple, their application is not always easy. Even with a good teacher, the force of habit often seems overwhelming. Instinctive, unreasoned direction is doggedly persistent and powerful. In comparison the dynamics of the Technique are so subtle that they can often be missed.

The Alexander Technique requires a true faith in reason, one that is often difficult to keep, particularly in the face of the confusion that inevitably accompanies personal transformation. The change that the Technique seeks is fundamental. It involves giving up our most intimate and comfortable habits and taking increasing responsibility for ourselves. This is not easy. As Alexander once said to a pupil, 'All that's worrying you is that what I ask you to do will bring about what I tell you it will bring about.'

The Technique presents a formidable challenge to those of us who are used to getting results by 'trying harder'. At the same time, ideas such as inhibition and attention to the means-whereby are easily misunderstood and misapplied. One must find the delicate balance between ends and means, control and spontaneity, doing and non-doing. This problem of balance is expressed in the paradox which is the heart of the Technique: 'give up trying too hard, but never give up'. One has to be patient and persevering. It is not a quick or easy process. The art of psychophysical balance requires nothing less than what Dewey called 'a revolution in thought and action'.

Education
for use

*Give a child conscious control and you
give him poise, the essential starting-point
for education.*

The education of children in Great Britain and the United States
has evolved over the past century through the interplay of two
major philosophies, the 'traditional' and the 'progressive'. The
traditional approach is based on inculcating children with a
certain body of knowledge considered essential for their mental
development. This knowledge is presented, to use Dewey's term,
'from without' in a disciplined and highly structured manner.

Subjects are not necessarily related to one another, nor is any
emphasis placed on making the material 'relevant' to the student's
experience. The child's task is to absorb the knowledge and to
reproduce it in examinations; those unable to do this are labelled
failures.

The weaknesses of this approach have become increasingly
evident. The sheer speed of technological and scientific development makes much of the information received in school irrel-
evant or just plain wrong within even a few years. Such rapid
change and innovation requires individuals to be able to think for
themselves and adapt to different circumstances. The 'progressive' philosophy, based on the principle of education 'from
within', aims to fill this need. It sees the task of the school as the
creation of a free and relatively unstructured environment in
which children are encouraged to learn by themselves *through
direct experience whenever possible*. Emphasis is placed on the
process of learning rather than on the results. Subjects are related

to an overall picture so as to make them more meaningful.

As Dewey pointed out, the progressive approach is much more difficult to implement than the traditional one. It is less mechanistic and requires more adaptability and creativity on the part of the teachers. Dewey recognized that the gap between progressive theory and practice could be traced to the confusion between external and internal freedoms and that numerous attempts at innovation had failed because discipline and order, which had previously been imposed by the system, were simply rejected outright. He emphasized that freedom from restraint and rigid structures is only the beginning. The progressive teacher must find a way of developing, in both herself and her pupils, the inner freedom that is an essential part of her work. Because inner freedom finds its expression in self-discipline it obviates the need for the gross imposition of discipline and order.

To apply these ideals on a large scale is an enormously complex task which requires radical change in the nature of our society. Nevertheless it is possible for an individual to begin to explore the meaning of inner freedom and its importance in education.

The Alexander Technique is one practical method by which this exploration can begin. Indeed some people have had great hopes for it. In his article 'Endgaining and Means Whereby' Huxley writes of Alexander's work:

> It is now possible to conceive of a totally new type of education affecting the entire range of human activity, from the physiological, through the intellectual, moral, and practical, to the spiritual – an education which by teaching them the proper use of the self, would preserve children and adults from most of the diseases and evil habits that now afflict them; an education whose training in inhibition and conscious control would provide men and women with the psychophysical means for behaving rationally and morally.[44]

This new type of education which Huxley describes is of course easier to conceive than to put into practice. There have, however, been a number of attempts to turn these ideals into a reality. The first was made under Alexander's direction by Irene Tasker, who in 1924 opened the first school to apply Alexander's principles to daily activities. After visiting her school Dewey wrote:

> I feel I am doing a public educational service in stating my judgement as to the great, even extraordinary value of her work. Miss Tasker is an experienced teacher with a natural gift for dealing with children. In addition, she is a thorough mistress of the principles, methods and technique of Mr Alexander's work. Any child committed to her care will be sure of achieving intellectual, and moral as well as physical improvement.[45]

Tasker took a special interest in children because she felt they were relatively free from fixed habits and had, in her own words, 'less to unlearn'. Many of her pupils had special disabilities such as flat feet, rounded shoulders, defective speech, inability to concentrate and mild retardation. Whatever the specific problem, Tasker always found that the child's general Use was at least to some extent misdirected and rather than concentrate on the disability, she devoted her energies to improving his Use. As she put it, she would teach the child 'how to prevent the misdirection of his use and help him, through making an improvement in the working of his primary control, to maintain a better use of himself as a whole in everything he does'.[46] This was because she had found that 'during the process of improvement in the child's use a corresponding improvement in his general functioning and in the quality of his output' took place. At the same time his specific disability tended gradually to disappear.

Although Tasker found it necessary to give children with special difficulties private attention outside daily classes, she also successfully taught children with comparatively good Use in groups. Indeed, she rarely taught the Technique individually in the classroom, concentrating on introducing the process of inhibition and direction through her own example and through group discussion and practice.

A specific example of Tasker's teaching method may help to illuminate her general approach. In an article in *The Alexander Journal*, Joyce Warrack relates that during preparations for the end of term play the children learnt the whole play resting on their backs and practising the directions for maintaining good Use. Emphasis was placed on inhibiting any immediate reaction to noise or interruption. This work went on for most of the term, during which problems of dramatic interpretation and expression were thoroughly considered. Two weeks or so before the performance the children started to rehearse. By this time they were so confident that the producer had virtually nothing more to do. One especially telling incident occurred during an outdoor production of *A Midsummer Night's Dream*:

> A noisy plane circled low over the garden, completely drowning the actors' voices. The small Titania was quite unperturbed and, with her finger to her lips, held the situation for three solid minutes till the intruder had flown off – then the play resumed quite calmly as if nothing had happened.[47]

Warrack gives another example of Alexander's principles in action, this time in a singing class. Tasker impressed upon the children that it was primarily a *listening* class. She began by singing a simple tune while the children practised inhibition and direction. Then she asked them to cross the floor and to sing the tune to her when they felt fully confident. For the first two classes no one did so. During the third class one child came and sang the melody effortlessly and was quickly followed by several others. External rewards were not used, and those children who did not feel ready to sing were not made to feel uncomfortable. 'By the end of the term the children were happily singing several unison songs in perfect tune...'

Joyce Roberts, a fine Alexander teacher in her own right, made the following comments after observing Tasker's class:

> Alexander's Technique was applied to... sitting, speaking, rising to perform some ordinary task. The pupils were of all ages from five years, and many of them were handicapped by serious problems, but the concentration, self-control and awareness they displayed were awe-inspiring. Each individual really was able, when called upon, to stop that disastrous

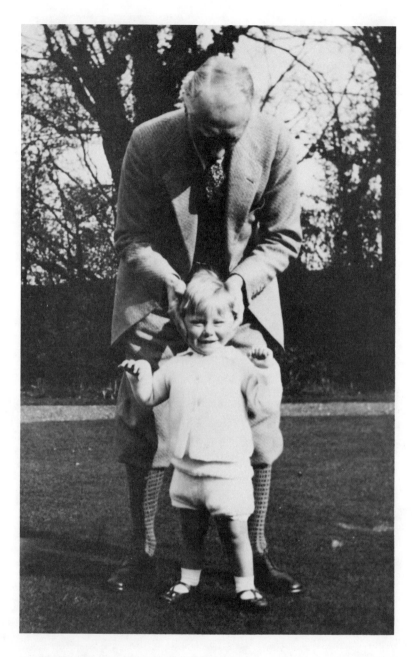

Alexander had a special love for children, and felt that his work should really be education, not re-education.

As he works on this infant he uses his hands delicately and skilfully to affirm the natural good Use the child shows. He is directing the infant's movements while supporting his tendency to upward expansion and freedom.

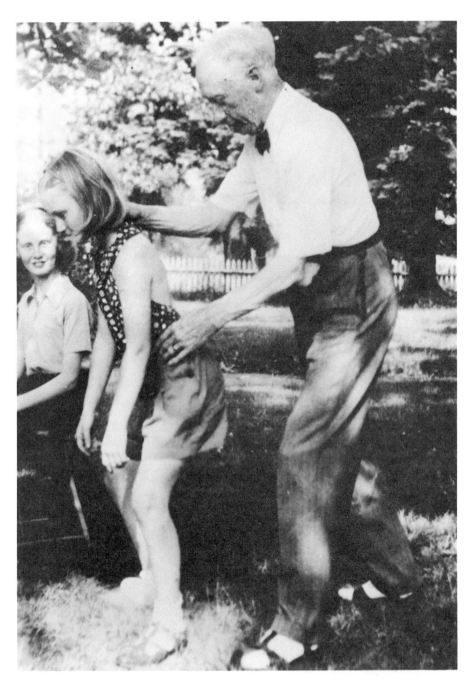

Here Alexander is assisting the young girl in bending while keeping her length. This lengthening allows the surfaces of the joints to separate infinitesimally, thus freeing up the movement. As she moves into bending Alexander encourages an integrated expansion in her whole body. This effect is achieved through using himself in a similar way and letting that good Use be communicated through his hands. 'Practise what you preach' is an essential rule for a teacher of the Alexander Technique.

immediate reaction to a stimulus – to think out a means-whereby, to wait until there was a perfectly clear picture in the mind as to what was required, and then with quiet confidence to let it happen. Onlookers caught a glimpse then of what that individual was capable of – what were the potentialities locked up, waiting to be released and developed.[48]

When I met Margaret Goldie, another pioneer teacher of the Alexander Technique, the impressions I had received of the work of Irene Tasker were confirmed and extended. Goldie spoke, with a quiet conviction born of over forty years' experience, of the importance of making the psychophysical integrity of the child the primary consideration in education. She specially emphasized Alexander's belief that 'the end for which they [the children] are working is of minor importance as compared with the way they direct the use of themselves for the gaining of that end', and pointed out that if this principle were adhered to the child would not only be happier and better balanced but that his school work would also be of a higher standard.

Goldie cited numerous examples from her own experience. One I particularly remember concerned a nine-year-old boy and his reactions to a problem in Latin. Goldie noticed from the manifestations of the child's Use that he was in difficulties. The boy explained that he could not manage the exercise he had been set. Without mentioning the exercise at all, she reminded him to attend to his own balance and inner state. After regaining his poise, the child quickly solved his problem. Goldie also mentioned further examples of the same principle applied to all aspects of the curriculum. These, she pointed out, were merely dramatic illustrations of the general effectiveness of the Technique in helping children to use their potential. All this does not deny that individual subjects must be well taught – there is no substitute for technical understanding. The issue is one of priorities. By attending to oneself first, as the child with the Latin problem demonstrated, the vicious circle of misuse/failure – misuse/failure can be stopped at its source.

An example from my own experience of working with children may help to clarify this point. An eight-year-old boy with

117

poor coordination was sent to me for help. Although he was very bright and a talented musician, he was constantly ridiculed at school because he was no good at games and, in particular, because he was quite unable to catch a ball. I did not need to look far for an explanation. The first time I saw him try to catch a ball he went into a pronounced startle pattern, pulling his head back, closing his eyes and flailing his arms. His reaction to ridicule at his lack of natural aptitude was to become yet more afraid. As his fear increased his Use of himself in this particular activity became worse, as did his actual performance. (This is the cycle of misuse/failure – misuse/failure to which I have already referred.) After giving him one or two fairly conventional lessons, I adopted a more radical approach. I stood on the opposite side of the room from him with a ball in my hands and asked him to stand still and look at me while putting his attention on the feeling of his feet on the floor and the easy balance of his head on his neck. When he was able to stand in a poised manner I threw the ball past him, having asked him not to respond to it but to maintain his own poise. At first he found this very difficult and jerked his head back as soon as the ball left my hands. Then I decided to play a game with him in which I counted to three before throwing; on three I would either throw or fake a throw. He often jumped when I pretended to throw. This enabled him to notice how he was preparing to catch, and he was even able to laugh at being caught out in this way. Soon he was able to stand quietly as the ball whizzed past him. The next step was for him to hold his hand out and let the ball bounce off it without trying to catch it and without flinching at all. We played the 'one-two-three' game with this exercise as well and he mastered it fairly quickly – and had a lot of fun at the same time! After this he tried to catch the ball, but only if it landed in his hands. We continued in this way and eventually he learnt to catch quite well. Then we went on successfully to work in the same way with throwing and kicking.

The vicious circle of misuse/failure *can* be stopped through attention to process. Good Use frees the body and mind to work in harmony. This is as true in 'mental' tasks (solving a Latin problem) as in 'physical' ones (catching a ball). Coordination of mind and body frees the child's innate capacity to learn. The aim of

Alexander's approach to education is to teach poise and to develop the capacity to choose. A child who learns these skills need not be 'bad' at anything. He will of course be better at some things than others, but if he is allowed to remain inwardly free he will learn more and enjoy more of whatever he does.

Applying these principles to an individual child is relatively easy in comparison with the challenge of working along these lines in schools. There has been only one large-scale attempt to apply Alexander's principles to the state school system. In England during the late 1960s and early 1970s Jack Fenton, a former headmaster of both primary and secondary schools and a lecturer in physical and health education at a teachers' training college, carried out an extensive research project involving over a thousand children. He provided teachers with an illustrated questionnaire to help them assess the standard of their pupils' kinaesthetic awareness and movement habits. The results showed that the majority of children had a poorly developed kinaesthetic sense and that most of them had inefficient habits of movement which tended to get worse over time.

Fenton attempted to make use of the methods of the Alexander Technique in dealing with these problems on a large scale. Projects were run at a number of primary and secondary schools for periods of up to six months. Their aim was to 'make pupils aware of the factors involved in acquiring and maintaining good use... to teach body mechanics in all situations and to develop a class or group approach to this subject which is preventative as well as re-educational'.[49]

Fenton was assisted by two qualified Alexander teachers. Each project began with seminars for the school teachers involved, designed to help them prepare for the introduction of the Technique into the curriculum. In most cases the Technique was introduced to the children by means of group work with the Alexander teachers during normal physical education classes, and discussions of anatomy and body mechanics in normal science classes. As the projects progressed, the theme of good and bad Use was explored in art and drama. The children drew pictures of activities being performed well and poorly, and cut out examples from magazine illustrations. They were also encouraged to practise 'miming' good and bad movement. The vast majority of teachers and children surveyed had almost no understanding of good movement. However, their work with the Technique gave the children a growing awareness that they did have a choice in the way they used themselves, and some of them, unlike their teachers, were able to change for the better simply by understanding how they were interfering with their natural functioning. Fenton found that children who received Alexander training often improved their classwork, 'no doubt through their greater ability to pay attention'. Those who received private attention because of special disabilities such as severe lordosis and stuttering also improved.

Fenton's book, *Choice of Habit*, and his film, *Better Use of the Body in Activity*, both contain a number of useful suggestions to help teachers to recognize and prevent the development of faulty habits of movement. Fenton also listed a number of factors that most teachers agreed helped to form bad habits, including carrying heavy books and bags; prolonged periods of sitting; unsuitable furniture; and boredom. He pointed out the harmful effects of many exercises done in routine physical education classes and emphasized the importance of eliminating activities that encourage compression of the spine and joint surfaces or otherwise restrict and limit movement. Mindless approaches to weight training, push-ups and other 'bodybuilding' techniques received special criticism.

My first direct experience of applying the Technique in schools came through my work with Jean Shepherd, a qualified Alexander teacher who has worked on a voluntary, informal basis with children at two very different schools. The first school I visited with her was in a suburban, white, working-class community in Essex. Arrangements for Jean to teach at the school had been made through the headmaster, who had taken private lessons and was enthusiastic about the Technique. At the time of my visit Jean had been working for one day a week with a class of eight-year-olds for several months. She taught small groups during free periods and children with special difficulties received individual attention. I assisted Jean with the small groups which concentrated on developing good Use in activities such as walking, reading, writing and sitting. I also gave juggling lessons to each of the groups and did a lecture-performance for the whole school.

The most vivid impression I gained was of the relative receptivity and openness of children when exposed to the Technique. The children we worked with were much more responsive than most adults; clearly habits were not as fixed. Most of them seemed capable of understanding and applying inhibition to their activities. They also appeared to enjoy working with the Technique. The effect of Jean's work on children with special disabilities was particularly striking. One little girl had a serious speech impediment. When she tried to speak, she would nuzzle her head towards her shoulder and produce virtually inaudible sounds. Jean worked with her for twenty minutes, emphasizing the means-whereby throughout. At the end of the session, smiling broadly and proud of herself, the child was reading poetry that could be heard across the room.

The other school I visited was in a poor, urban, multi-racial district of London. The arrangements for teaching were similar although the conditions in the school were very different. The first school had been modern, well-equipped and run on the 'open classroom' plan. This one, by contrast, was old and over-crowded and followed traditional methods. Jean was working here with a class of seven-year-olds. She attended to each child during the course of the morning and also gave brief lessons in reading and anatomy. The regular teacher was eager to cooperate and corrected the children's Use with the same diligence she applied to correcting their grammar and spelling. Demolition work outside and noise from other classrooms made conditions far from ideal. Yet Jean's work seemed to be effective, and our class became the quietest in the school.

In the autumn of 1978, I had the opportunity to participate in a 'stress alleviation project' in schools at Redhill, Surrey, sponsored by the Surrey Back Pain Association and coordinated by Susan Thame, an Alexander teacher with experience in both education and industry, assisted by Sophia Gordon-Dean. The project focused on two junior schools for children under nine years old, and one middle school, attended by children between nine and thirteen. Thame had spent the term before the project began observing classroom work and getting to know the staff. The project started officially when the three of us went together to each school to give a presentation and answer questions from the teachers. In the presentations we emphasized that our main concern was to provide a resource for the teachers themselves; it seemed pointless to attempt to teach children the principles of good Use unless they were provided with good examples and given encouragement and assistance from teachers who understood those principles.

After the initial presentation we were each assigned a school; mine was the middle school. I visited each class and afterwards discussed with the teacher the children's particular problems and ways in which we could work together to solve them. The teachers were also offered individual Alexander lessons. Some of the teachers refused to take lessons and were reluctant to do anything for themselves; they insisted that their job was to teach the children, and the only help they wanted was advice that could immediately be put into effect in the classroom. One teacher in particular epitomized this attitude. When I visited him in his classroom he handed me a typed list of stress problems and challenged me to write the answers in the space he had provided. The list described some very real problems: chair and desk size in relation to the children's varying shapes, overcrowding, noise, inadequate ventilation, poor lighting and so on. The one problem he did not list, however, was the most pressing – his own state. He was stiff and tense, his back was hunched, and he moved and spoke with strain. He was teaching poor Use to the children every day through his own example.

Ironically, those teachers who did take advantage of the individual lessons were those who needed them least. The headmaster confirmed this when he mentioned that only his best teachers seemed to be involving themselves. This was also the case at the other schools.

The project developed with a core of teachers and head teachers from each of the schools. Attempts were made to help teachers convey their understanding of the Technique in the classroom. There was a growing consensus among the teachers participating that they needed more intensive training in the Alexander Technique if they were to embody the principles they hoped to teach. Unfortunately the project was not able to continue because of lack of funds.

The Alexander approach to education is to encourage the development of self-awareness and responsibility through attention to the means-whereby. The present education system seems to work against this. Children are sent to school shortly after they begin to develop an independent ego or 'I'. The transition from the instinctive world of infancy to the emerging consciousness of childhood is crucial for the development of the individual. Yet at school children are subject to enormous pressure. We demand that they sit for much of the day; we emphasize achievement in reading and writing and in mathematics without paying enough attention to how children are using themselves in these activities. We look for results rather than successes. In this way we teach them to become endgainers. It is no wonder that bright and generally well-balanced five-year-olds often become tense and uncoordinated seven-year-olds. Indeed, just by requiring children to write we are providing a stimulus which can, and usually does, distort their coordination. Writing is a complex skill and, unlike speaking, it is not instinctive. It has to be consciously learned. The image of a child hunched over his desk, tongue protruding and fingers gripping the pencil or crayon is familiar to everyone. Indeed, one teacher in the Surrey project reported that she found impressions from a child's writing through twenty pages of his pad. Imagine the tension behind that pen.

Clearly something is wrong. How can we expect our children to use an instrument properly when we fail to teach them how to use themselves? And how can we teach them to use themselves properly when we ourselves rely on unconscious habit?

The 'traditional' approach to education placed great emphasis on posture training. Teachers were trained to correct their children's manner of sitting and to show them the proper way of holding a pen. This training was very crude, but although it is no longer taught nothing has been put in its place. The younger Surrey teachers were acutely aware of this critical blank spot in their training, and even the older ones agreed that their training was insufficient.

A classic example of this problem is described in a Master's thesis by Alexander teacher Ann Matthews, entitled 'Implications for Education in the Work of F.M. Alexander'. Matthews worked with teachers and students in a school in New York State and she writes:

> A teacher calls her six- and seven-year-olds to gather round her on the floor and listen to a story. Most sit cross-legged with their spines collapsed into a curve and their heads pulled back onto their necks as they look up at the teacher. One boy is kneeling close to the teacher, back beautifully aligned, head balancing on the top. 'Thomas, you are blocking the people behind you,' says the teacher in a reproachful tone. 'Sit down so they can see the pictures.' The child sits down obediently and collapses like the others around him. The teacher does not see... that she has required the child to go from a poised, balanced, alert position, to one that is cramped and distorted. Knowing better than to protest, the child looks resigned.

It is clear to me from my work in schools and with a few committed teachers that the state education system does not at present adequately help children to develop from a condition of instinctive guidance to one of conscious control. At the same time, my experiences have helped to bring to life many of the inspiring ideas put forward by the early teachers of the Alexander Technique. The most sensible application is not in re-education but in prevention. As Dewey writes:

> [Alexander's] discovery could not have been made and the method of procedure perfected except by dealing with adults who were badly coordinated. But the method is not one of remedy; it is one of constructive education. Its proper field of application is with the young, with the growing generation, in order that they may come to possess as early as possible in life a correct standard of sensory appreciation and self-judgement. When once a reasonably adequate part of a

new generation has become properly coordinated, we shall have assurance for the first time that men and women in the future will be able to stand on their own feet, equipped with satisfactory psycho-physical equilibrium, to meet with readiness, confidence, and happiness instead of with fear, confusion and discontent, the buffetings and contingencies of their surroundings.[50]

Dewey and Alexander both believed that education should be devoted to the development of individual responsibility and freedom from mindless habit. They both realized that the demands of modern life could not be met by children merely with a command of facts but rather by individuals educated to command themselves.

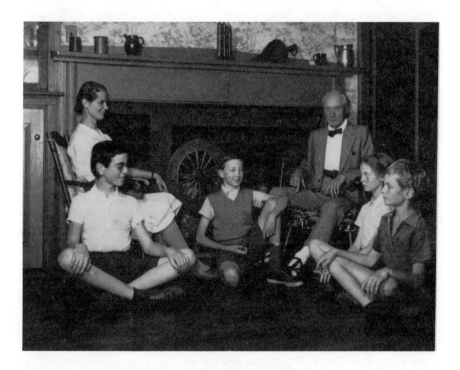

I love this photo of Alexander with children

What can I
do myself?

*We can throw away the habits of a lifetime in a
few minutes if we use our brains.*

A number of books published recently have tried to put forward a 'do-it-yourself' method of learning the Alexander Technique. One claims to show how easy it is to learn the Technique, another reveals a set of 'secret Alexander exercises'. With or without a book, there is no way of learning how to 'do' the Alexander Technique, because the Technique is not concerned with doing but with *undoing*; and there are, of course, no secret exercises.

Alexander's own answer to those who wrote to him for advice was to remind them that new sensory experiences could not be gained by written or spoken words alone. Any attempt to develop new Use, to 'get it right', by direct action is doomed to failure; the process approach rather than the habitual one of 'endgaining' must be followed and must be combined with an attitude of openness to the unknown and a willingness to suspend the judgements conveyed by 'feelings'.

Although with a teacher you can learn in a matter of a few weeks what it took Alexander years to attain, any attempt to apply Alexander's principles and practice *without* guidance can provide a valuable and rapid lesson in humility! It is, however, possible to begin to increase your self-awareness and to deepen your understanding of the Use of the self by practising the art of observation.

Start right now by becoming aware of what you are doing as you read this book. Can you notice any unnecessary tension in your fingers, hands, arms, shoulders, neck, stomach, hips, legs, face or eyes? Is your body in a balanced alignment? Questions such as these are difficult to answer due to the distorting effects of unreliable sensory appreciation. In order to get a clearer sense of how we use ourselves it helps to have objective points of reference. One of these is, of course, the mirror.

In order to make effective use of the mirror, or any other form of feedback, we have to learn to avoid making value judgements. The habit of labelling everything as good or bad, right or wrong, attractive or unattractive is associated with a deep pattern of tension and misuse. We can begin to free ourselves from this pattern by simply looking at and accepting what *is*: this is the first step towards real change.

Stand in front of a mirror and just look for a few minutes. Don't adjust your shirt or brush your hair – just look. Then see if you can tell to which side your head is leaning. Is one shoulder higher than the other? If you look carefully you will probably be able to see that one shoulder *is* higher and tighter than the other and that the head is tilted very slightly away from the lower shoulder. You may find yourself wanting to correct what you see by holding your head straight and dropping the higher shoulder. Any attempt to do this will, however, result in the creation of a compensatory maladjustment, in the substitution of one pattern of overtension for another. Integration results not from specific, direct actions but rather from an indirect approach which at all times considers the balance of the whole.

If you now compare the two sides of your body, you can begin to observe the effects of habitual Use on structure. The dominant side – usually the right, just as most people are right-handed – tends to be more developed and the torso often twists towards the less dominant side. Notice how the different parts of your body relate to one another. In most people the head, rib-cage and pelvis are out of alignment and the body as a whole appears either to be pulled down by gravity or held up tightly to resist it.

I have emphasized throughout this book the key role that the head and neck play in integrating all parts of the body. The first step towards gaining a practical understanding of this role is to find out exactly where your head balances on your neck. Using the tips of your index fingers, point to the place where you think your head rests on your spine. Most people place their fingers much too low; the balance point is located in the hollow under the ear lobe.

Another important area with which most of us are unfamiliar is that of the hip joints. Bend down and pick up something from the floor. Then place your index fingers at the point from which you bend your torso. Most people put their fingers at the top of the pelvic girdle rather than at the actual hip joint. In fact the hip joints are much lower than most of us think. The common habit of bending from the waist breaks the integrity of the spine and deadens our kinaesthetic sense.

An understanding of the workings of all the joints is crucial to good Use of the self. Our joints not only make movement possible, they are also centres of our kinaesthetic feedback system. If a joint is misused the kinaesthetic information coming from it to the brain will be distorted, leading to further misuse. The simple fact is that the majority of us do not know where any of the major joints of the body are located, and we misuse ourselves accordingly.

Still in front of the mirror, go on to explore the exact location and range of movements of all the joints, remembering that they always work as part of a whole system. You may find it helpful to consult a simple anatomy text or even a model skeleton. Practical knowledge of basic anatomy and body mechanics will help you in making more accurate observations about what you do with yourself and will give you clues about what not to do.

We can also gain valuable information about ourselves from the surfaces we touch. You can observe yourself by becoming aware of all the contact points of your body against the surfaces you are touching: the chair, the floor, and so on. You can get information not only about those things but about yourself as well. Try lying face down on the floor (not on the bed – the surface must be hard if you are to get accurate feedback) with your arms close to your body and your hands at your sides, palms facing upwards. Now turn your head to the side and just rest. Allow yourself to appreciate the security of this position: you cannot fall, the body is completely supported and you can let go of all the tensions that you normally think you need to hold yourself up. If you stay still for several minutes you will be able to notice a more appropriate distribution of tension in your body. Muscles that are habitually tense will begin to release and you will feel an increasing contact with the floor. It is interesting at this point to compare what you noticed in the mirror about the two sides of the body with what the floor is telling you.

Lying prone on the floor is just one of the numerous methods available for producing a state of relaxation. The problem with this and other methods comes when we begin to move, and our habitual tensions reassert themselves. What is needed is a means for achieving relaxation in action.

Having achieved a degree of relaxation you must now consider standing up again. Notice how you make the transition from the thought of moving to the movement itself. Can you detect a preparatory pattern of tension when you first consider moving? Most people will tense the neck, shoulders, lower back and hamstrings as soon as the very idea of making a movement occurs to them. See if you can move with fewer preparatory tensions. First of all, move into a crawling position. Then wait. Now move into an upright posture.

Congratulations! You have just re-enacted a process that took millions of years of evolution to develop. The fully upright posture is much less stable than any quadrupedal disposition. It creates the possibility of effortless, easy movement but at the same time can cause tremendous insecurity if it is not functioning properly. Unfortunately, most of us chronically interfere with our balance by working too hard to hold ourselves up.

This overworking is extremely difficult to notice because it takes place below consciousness and conditions our sensory appreciation. It is possible, however, to increase one's awareness of the play of balance. Stand in front of the mirror again, with your weight evenly distributed on both feet. Take off your shoes in order to get the maximum feedback from the floor. If you stand 'still' for three or four minutes you will start to notice the subtle shifts and adjustments of tension that are taking place. (You may want to reflect on how rarely you stand on two feet with your weight evenly distributed. It is unusual to see anyone who is not constantly shifting his weight from one leg to the other or leaning against something in order to stay up.) By raising one leg off the ground, you will get a clearer experience of your balance at work.

Now, still standing on one leg, close your eyes. When you begin to lose your balance notice what happens – most people pull their heads back and tense up.

If you wish to explore this question of balance further, I recommend that you get hold of a long 2" x 4" (5cm x 10cm) piece of wood (or a balance beam if one is available) and practise walking on it, first with eyes open and then with eyes closed. If you succeed in mastering this, you're ready to try a tightrope or unicycle!

The quality of your voice and breathing is another valuable point of reference for self-observation. Start reading out loud at the top of this page and listen to the sound of your voice. After you have read a few paragraphs, deliberately pull your head back and notice the change in the quality of your voice. This is a crude but effective way of observing the effect of Use on functioning. To investigate this relationship further it helps to have some standard of comparison. Take a line of verse or, more simply, a whispered vowel sound such as aaaaahhhhh, and repeat it occasionally while engaged in any day-to-day activity. Listen to the quality of tone, noticing whether it is fluid or broken. The way you use yourself will determine the ease with which the sound flows.

When you study your breathing, remember that the purpose is to increase your awareness of the effects of Use on functioning. Never try to change or improve your breathing directly. Like circulation and digestion, breathing is a natural function, and the only way it can be improved is to create the right conditions in the whole organism by changing unnecessary tension patterns within the body that interfere with it. If you brace your knees back for twenty seconds and notice the effects on your diaphragm and breathing, you will get an idea of how these patterns operate.

Now, bearing all this in mind, stand quietly and observe your breathing. Follow the flow of air in through the nostrils and out again – don't try to influence it in any way, just listen in as detached a manner as possible. Then observe what you do with your neck, shoulders, rib-cage, pelvis and knees as you breathe. Notice how the rhythm changes when you begin to move. Direct your attention to your breathing in various activities such as lifting, speaking, running and meeting someone new. Note particularly the things that make you hold your breath.

Observing others can provide a valuable source of information for your study. If you can observe *without criticizing* you can learn a great deal. Look at people in everyday situations: on the street, at home, in the office. How do they use themselves? Do they appear to be flowing up or pulled down? Observe the use of their joints, paying particular attention to the way the head is balanced. Try to get a sense of the distribution of tension, noting which parts of their bodies are stiff and which collapsed. Look at typists, dentists, carpenters, musicians: can you see how their lives have shaped their bodies? Look at people whom you consider to be examples of grace and poise: perhaps a favourite entertainer or sportsman. Notice what they do *not* do with themselves. And look at your parents. Is your posture and movement pattern like theirs? And is your children's like yours?

The most important area of observation is the nature and speed of your reactions. Many of us experience a sense of being 'on edge' or jumpy. This is really a habitual over-reaction to our environment. One way of deepening your understanding of this is to experiment with habitual patterns of reacting to a familiar stimulus, such as a door-bell or a telephone ringing. You may have noticed that you tend to 'jump' at these noises. Next time, see if you can pause, just for two seconds, before reaching for the telephone or getting up to answer the door. Remember, however, that to pause properly does not mean interfering with your breathing or tensing up before you move. Try to remain perfectly still without being fixed in any way. When you have practised this for some time, try to do the same thing when someone asks you a question or calls your name.

Most of these observation exercises turn out to be extremely difficult because so often we rely on our habits to study our habits. Indeed, their greatest value is in increasing our awareness of the power of habit. But, you might ask, why bother about these everyday habits? Most of us manage to get through each day without paying them much attention, and we all have problems that seem much more pressing than how we use ourselves. My reply is that, more than the big events – the traumas and the ecstasies – it is the choice we make about the way we conduct ourselves every day that determines the quality of our lives.

Further adventures in learning how to learn

In the years since *Body Learning* was originally published I have made my living primarily by travelling around the world, leading seminars on learning how to learn. Throughout this time I have regularly challenged myself to learn new things. In addition to enriching my life, these learning challenges keep my work fresh by deepening my insight into the process of learning. Each of these endeavours has further confirmed and extended my understanding of the value of the Alexander Technique. Let me describe some of them for you:

Learning to swim

When I was seven years old my counsellors at summer camp threw me into the deep end of the lake in a misguided attempt to help me overcome my terror of deep water and swimming in general. Of course, their intervention had the opposite effect.

When I was twelve my parents sent me for swimming lessons with a kind, patient teacher. I learned to swim reasonably well in shallow water. In the last lesson the teacher invited me to dive off the diving board into the deepest part of the pool. Although I was still frightened, his encouragement drove me on and I leapt into the water. After this my fear seemed to recede. I wouldn't say that I actually enjoyed swimming, but I no longer went out of my way to avoid it. Occasionally I would go swimming and usually found that although I could swim rapidly (I was still highly motivated to get out of the deep water by getting to the other side of the pool as fast as possible!), my stamina, which was considerable on land, was virtually non-existent in the water. I generally had to rest between laps and rarely swam for more than five or ten minutes.

In the early 1980s I decided to apply my understanding of the Alexander Technique to improve both my stamina and my level of enjoyment in the water. I was fortunate to have as my swimming coach one of the world's greatest teachers, Tony Buzan. In addition to his expertise in applying brain research to accelerate learning, Buzan was a superb swimmer who had received Olympic level coaching. He was also one of my most perspicacious Alexander students.

At my first lesson, Tony noticed that despite my status as a successful Alexander teacher I was pulling my head back ferociously while swimming. The old fear was so strong that it overrode my conscious intention. Tony suggested that I move to the shallow end of the pool and practice breathing while holding on to the side.

He suggested that I think about 'making friends with the water' as I inhibited my tendency to contract my neck muscles, while directing toward an overall lengthening and widening. With a little practice I was able to maintain a new, freer use of myself in the shallow end. Next I graduated to swimming widths of the pool across the shallow end. I found that as I let my neck be free, my arms and legs freed up considerably and I began to glide through the water in what felt like an effortless fashion. After a few weeks of practice I was ready for the deep end. Tony suggested that I direct my head toward the opposite end of the pool and let my body follow, extending my arms and kicking my legs from the hip. When I began to tighten up and get short of breath, I would pause at the side of the pool and give myself directions for the free and easy use of my head and neck. When I felt confident that I could sustain the directions for improved use in action, I would launch back into my laps. After a little practice my swimming had improved dramatically. I could do three or four laps without tiring and, best of all, I really began to enjoy it.

For the next few years I practised swimming whenever I could, applying Alexander principles. I taught myself to turn my head to alternate sides to make my swimming 'ambidextrous' and learned the butterfly and breaststrokes. In 1984, I passed a major milestone, achieving something I never would have thought possible when I was a child – I swam a mile. Actually I swam a mile plus one extra lap just to celebrate that I wasn't too tired. It was one of the most exhilarating moments of my life and, once again, F.M. Alexander played a key role in making it possible!

Learning to lead seminars and give speeches

In 1978 I began to travel around the world leading seminars in psychophysical re-education. Since then I have spent an average of a hundred days a year teaching and speaking to groups ranging from senior corporate executives and military officers to school teachers and physicians. My presentations vary from one hour keynote addresses and after-dinner speeches to five-day intensive residential programmes. The audiences range in size from six to more than ten thousand people. It is not unusual for me to spend eight or more hours a day speaking. Despite this frequently gruelling schedule I have never suffered from laryngitis or lost my voice. But the Alexander Technique offers much more than just a means of preserving the vocal mechanism under stress: it reveals the inner secrets that allow fear and stage fright to be transformed into confidence and enthusiasm; it awakens a sense of poise that translates into a commanding presence.

For the first few years of my speaking career, I was usually the youngest person in the room. Most of my speaking and teaching engagements were with senior level business people and in those days I did not know much about business. It would have been very easy to be intimidated, especially when faced with the challenging questions with which I was often greeted. When faced with a hostile question or sceptical look, I was prone to two types of automatic responses: I felt like either shrinking up and disappearing or puffing up my chest and taking the offensive. Applying the Alexander Technique allowed me to 'stand my ground': I was generally able to inhibit both of these tendencies, look the person square in the eye and give a reasoned answer.

Over the years I have given presentations in a number of challenging and stressful situations. I have addressed royalty, heads of state, impatient executives, cynical employees and 'juvenile deliquents'. I once auditioned for a series of speaking engagements that would represent one third of my annual income. And I've been interviewed by all manner of media, including my first-ever appearance on an American radio show, which began with the greeting, 'You're in the hot seat and you're on the air!' Yet each time, through the application of Alexander's principles, I was able to prevent the pattern of contraction inspired habitually by such circumstances. Although I felt serious 'butterflies in the stomach', the application of inhibition and direction trained the butterflies to 'fly in formation'. Fear and stage fright metamorphosed into positive energy and enthusiasm.

The Alexander Technique is more than just a means of preserving the voice, avoiding intimidation and coping with stage fright. It has taught me to prevent interference with my natural poise on stage, to *be* fully with an audience, and to enjoy it.

Learning aikido

When I was a youngster I was fascinated by the grace and power of martial arts. I watched Bruce Lee move like a tiger and admired David Carradine's wizardry as he effortlessly resolved conflict in *Kung Fu*. In 1975, while training as a teacher of the Alexander Technique, I saw my first demonstration of the art of aikido. Whirling and spinning like a top, a diminutive Japanese man tossed much bigger attackers around like juggling balls.

Aikido, literally translated as 'the way of harmonious energy', is a Japanese martial art developed by Morihei Ueshiba (1883–1969). It is based on moving and breathing in harmony with an attacking force. Rather than trying to disable or destroy an opponent, the aikidoist uses the energy of an attack to imbalance or immobilize an aggressor without causing injury.

As the years passed I read a number of books about aikido, attended more demonstrations and endeavoured to apply the aikido philosophies of 'centering' and 'blending with conflict' in my personal and professional life. I daydreamed about the possibility of mastering the art but never made the commitment to put in the time and effort necessary to learn. Then, when I was 35, I did an exercise which I recommended to all my students – I imagined myself on my death bed looking back at my life wondering: what would I regret not having done? The answer was clear: learning the art of aikido!

Shortly thereafter I attended a seven-day intensive aikido camp. I found a school and a superb master near my home in Washington DC and sought out local aikido clubs in my travels. I made a personal commitment to attain a black belt rank before my fortieth birthday and to use my study of aikido to deepen my understanding of the Alexander work.

The first challenge was to my ego. I was used to being in charge of groups, to teaching others how to think and move. Big companies paid me considerable sums to talk about mind–body coordination and poise. Yet, when I walked on to the aikido mat with my stiff new uniform and pristine white belt, I was clearly at the bottom of the totem pole. Even more humiliating, when I attempted to execute aikido techniques I was regularly reminded by my teacher and senior students to 'try to be more upright' and 'not try so hard'.

Despite being hoisted regularly with my own petard, I persevered. My years of experience with the Alexander work taught me that learning involves 'going from the known to the unknown', that learning something new requires unlearning something old. After a few months of familiarizing myself with the Japanese names for the techniques and learning how to fall, I realized that the main challenge of learning aikido would be to *inhibit fearful or aggressive responses* to the stimuli provided by the various attacks offered by my partners.

After training seven days a week for almost four years, I went up for my black belt test. It proved to be an exhilarating celebration of inhibition and direction. Throughout the test I felt like I was standing in the eye of a hurricane, the quiet centre of a storm of attacks. It was even more fun than juggling.

I gained my black belt. The Japanese word for black belt is *shodan* which means 'first step' or 'certified beginner'. With Alexander's help I fulfilled my childhood dream and entered my forties as a certified beginner!

4

The Questing Spirit

*Light, seeking light, doth light of
light beguile.*

WILLIAM SHAKESPEARE,
Love's Labour Lost, 1.i.

The Alexander
work and
organizational
change

After a few years of conducting seminars, I noticed that while
the individuals in my classes reported considerable benefits, the
organizations in which they worked remained fundamentally
unchanged. The environments and 'cultures' of many of these
organizations simply were not conducive to learning, creative
thinking and personal fulfilment. It dawned on me that individual development must be promoted in the context of organizational development.

At the same time, global competition was beginning to force
many organizations to change. Top-heavy, unwieldy bureaucracies tried to become responsive and agile overnight. Corporate
leaders started preaching the necessity of continuous improvement, personal accountability, risk-taking and 'empowerment'.
Individuals were challenged to learn new technologies and organizational systems faster than ever before. With fewer people
and more to do, stress levels began rising to new heights.

This whirlwind of change has accelerated in recent years.
Facilitating this organizational evolution is a complex and challenging job. My clients find that the application of Alexander's
principles provides an invaluable compass by which to navigate
amid chaos. Here are just a few of the ways that Alexander's
'operational ideas' are relevant to organizations.

Use and functioning

The word corporation comes from the root 'corpus' meaning 'body'. Most corporate bodies suffer, writ large, from the same unreasoned habits and lack of conscious control that plague individuals. Many organizations are compelled, for example, by fear-inspired habit, toward a short-term, exploitative, unsound approach to doing business. And, believe it or not, these organizations continue to operate in this way not so much out of evil but from ignorance. They do not recognize that they, in Alexander terms, have a choice about how to use themselves.

The first step in organizational change is questioning habitual modes of operation while recognizing that choice is possible.

The whole person

Alexander emphasized that 'the human organism always functions as a whole and can only be fundamentally changed as a whole'. The same is true of organizations. As the complexity of our world multiplies exponentially, the application of 'systems thinking' becomes more urgent. Organizational consultant Peter Senge, author of *The Fifth Discipline* (see Bibliography, page 174), defines systems thinking as 'seeing interrelationships rather than linear cause and effect chains and seeing processes of change rather than snapshots'. He argues that 'the unhealthiness of our world today is in direct proportion to our inability to see it as a whole.'

Experience of the Alexander work makes one much more intimately attuned to the perception and management of the whole.

Primary Control

In the individual, the Primary Control is the point of greatest leverage for organizing the system into a coordinated whole. The 'head' of an organization functions analogously.

Organizations will be coordinated to the extent that their senior management encourages and actively supports universal participation in clarifying and living humane, systems-oriented visions, missions and values. When leaders 'walk their talk' they nurture a shared sense of purpose that integrates and coordinates the action of all their members.

Total, unwavering commitment by senior management is the

first step, the Primary Control, in the process of organizational change and development.

Unreliable sensory appreciation

Most big organizations began life as an expression of an idealistic vision of one extraordinary person. As the organization grows it almost invariably falls prey to bureaucratic habits, and idealism falls by the wayside.

Then rapid changes force bureaucracies to try to return to their more creative, entrepreneurial roots. Massive efforts are made to change cultures, to promote leadership, quality, risk-taking and empowerment. Many senior managers travel around giving 'motivational' talks on change while continuing to function in a bureaucratic mode. They are usually unaware that their behaviour is out of alignment with their words.

Alexander became aware that he couldn't be sure he was doing what he thought he was doing while attempting to change a habit. The same is true for people in organizations. Alexander's work provides a model for individuals and organizations to question the reliability of their perceptions so they are more likely to make the translation from 'idealistic theory into actual practice'.

Inhibition

Alexander said that for the right thing to happen one had first to stop doing the wrong thing. As individuals learn to question their bureaucratic, hierarchical world-view they can choose not to act it out. Many organizations, for example, are hungry for new approaches to creative thinking and problem solving. But progress in this area is elusive without recognizing that, as William James emphasized, 'Genius... means little more than the faculty of perceiving in a non-habitual way.'

For individuals and organizations, inhibition is the corner-stone of change.

Direction

Inhibition sets the stage for direction. When old habits are made conscious and a delay is interposed between a stimulus and the habitual response, something new can happen.

The organizational equivalent of direction (neck to be free, head forward and up, etc.) is systems-oriented strategic planning in the context of a shared sense of vision, mission and values.

An organization will be successful to the extent to which its members consciously integrate its vision, mission, plan and values in their daily lives.

Ends and means

The extraordinary growth of Japan's economy since World War II has been greatly influenced by an approach to business called Total Quality Management or 'TQM'. Curiously, this approach was pioneered by an American, Dr W. Edwards Deming. Western companies ignored Deming's advice after the war so he went to Japan where he became a hero.

Now, in Britain, the United States and around the world, organizations are urgently attempting to reform themselves in accordance with Deming's principles. Management guru and bestselling author Stephen Covey sums up the essence of TQM thus: '... quality, the result, is a function of quality, the process.'

Alexander's work offers a profound, process-oriented approach to improving the quality of life and of performance. Alexander invited us to 'continually improve' the process we apply in achieving our goals. The success of the quality revolution requires the application of Alexander's emphasis on 'means-whereby' ('quality, the process') to business operations.

The bottom line: freedom from fear

To achieve quality, organizations must, according to Deming, 'drive out fear.' He emphasizes that fear prevents people from acknowledging mistakes and asking for help, making continuous improvement impossible. 'The economic loss from fear,' he writes, 'is appalling.'

Habits of responding fearfully run deep. The Alexander work offers a practical method for freeing ourselves from the legacy of fear. This freedom supports individual fulfilment and organizational success. Although it is not a panacea, the Alexander Technique does offer a profound experience of quality from the inside out – an experience which often provides the missing link in efforts to change.

Alexander questions and answers

Since *Body Learning* first appeared I have been asked many questions by students around the world. Here are some of the most frequent and most interesting questions, with my replies:

How many lessons will I need?

How long does it take to learn to play the guitar? How many lessons are needed to learn to speak Japanese? Obviously, it depends upon your purpose. Do you want to be the next Segovia or Clapton, or just to play a few simple tunes? Do you intend to translate haiku, or are you simply preparing for a two-week vacation? Although the skill of your teacher and your talent level will certainly influence your progress, the duration and intensity of your study will be determined ultimately by the level of expertise that you seek.

Just like learning a musical instrument or a new language, the number of Alexander lessons you need will vary in accordance with your purpose. Pupils who come for relief of physical problems often stop lessons when their pain disappears, and this can sometimes happen in the first few sessions. To keep it from returning, however, they will probably need more lessons. Musicians, singers, actors, athletes and others interested in performance-improvement frequently find that they continue to benefit from long-term study. I've had some students learn a tremendous amount and make great changes from just one lesson, while others have had thirty or more without changing as much.

Alexander suggested that a basic course of thirty lessons was necessary for an individual to begin successfully applying the Technique on their own. Despite the individual differences, I've observed that, on average, the people who get the most from the Technique are those who begin with a fairly intensive programme of thirty to forty lessons.

How often should I come for lessons?

When I first studied the Alexander Technique in 1973, the prevailing wisdom was that the pupils should come for lessons as frequently as possible. The general prescription was to come four or five times the first week, three or four times for the next two weeks, and then twice a week until the thirty lessons were completed. The logic was that, to overcome the inertia of habit, one required an intensive experience to liberate new patterns of use. This intensive introduction is an alignment with the best understanding of effective adult learning. Concentrated practice in the early stages of an endeavour dramatically improves the value of future practice, whether in learning a language, learning to juggle or learning the Alexander Technique. Just as a spacecraft uses most of its fuel in take-off to break the earth's gravitational field, so the new student will benefit from an initial, intensive programme of realigning their relationship to gravity.

Although the 1970s were hectic, they now seem like halcyon days compared to the 1990s. Many of my prospective students are too stressed and too busy to study stress and time management. The demands of the modern calendar make it extraordinarily difficult for individuals to come for lessons more than once or twice a week. Nevertheless, I recommend that you have as many lessons as possible in your first few weeks of study. A good alternative is to attend one of the excellent weekend or week-long Alexander Technique retreats where you can immerse yourself in the work. You can begin your private lessons after this intensive introduction. Recommended weekend and week-long seminars can be found by writing to STAT or NASTAT (see Useful Addresses, page 178).

What actually happens in a lesson?

The essence of an Alexander lesson is a guided experience in improving coordination through application of inhibition and direction. Each teacher develops her own way of communicating these principles and the experience of improved use. Every pupil has his own way of learning and incorporating the principles.

Some teachers spend the first lesson getting to know the student, finding out why she's coming for lessons, and creating a verbal rapport before the 'hands-on' work begins. Other teachers say hello, ask you to stand in front of a chair, and get right to work.

Some teachers begin with an explanation of Alexander's discovery of the principles and perhaps a demonstration, using a skeleton or other anatomical teaching device. Other teachers trust that they can communicate most of the necessary information using their hands, a few words and a well-placed mirror.

Some teachers prefer to focus on helping students apply the principles to the simple acts of sitting, standing, walking, bending over or reaching to pick something up. Others prefer to work with their students resting on the floor or on the table to free them from any stimulus towards misuse.

Some teachers are keen to help their pupils apply the principles in more complex activities: from singing an aria, reciting a soliloquy or playing the violin to working on the computer, talking on the telephone or riding a horse.

Many teachers apply all of the above approaches, depending on the circumstances.

Whatever external activities are conducted in the lesson, you will be introduced to the application of inhibition and direction to learn a new, improved use of the self.

How do I know if I have found a good teacher?

Alexander emphasized that an 'efficient teacher of my principles' would combine the 'aptitudes and intuitions of an artist' with a 'special training and... [a] keen eye for character needed to detect and to eradicate the mental difficulties, and the vocal, respiratory and other physiological delusions which almost invariably accompany physical defects'.

• • •

How do you know if someone who calls themselves a teacher of the Alexander Technique has received the 'special training' and, more importantly, possesses the requisite skills to guide you?

Certification by the Society of Teachers of the Alexander Technique is a useful but not foolproof guide to finding a good teacher. Although there are some excellent teachers who are not certified and some poor teachers who are, generally, certified graduates of STAT and STAT-affiliated training courses (see listing in Useful Addresses, page 178) will be of a high standard.

Good Alexander teachers come in all shapes, sizes and styles but whatever their physical endowment they move with intelligence and economy of effort. Good Alexander teachers do not need perfect poise, but rather, sufficient experience in working on themselves to be able to guide others successfully. In addition to skill in using their hands to guide you toward improved Use, good Alexander teachers demonstrate the characteristics shared by good teachers in all disciplines: patience, compassion, humour, creativity and a commitment to bring out the best in you.

Use common sense in finding and evaluating a teacher. If someone is well-recommended by a friend or if their name appears on the STAT list, then give them a try. Always feel free to ask questions. You might ask, for example, how your teacher has benefited from the Technique or why they chose to become a teacher. Trust your intuition: if you do not feel a sense of rapport or trust, then try someone else.

Why do many teachers focus on the movement from sitting to standing?

Getting in and out of a chair is an everyday movement that provides a wealth of opportunity for learning. It requires the active participation of the major joints of the body and quickly reveals fundamental patterns of discoordination. Most people pull their heads back, shorten their stature and hold their breath while performing this simple act. Some Alexander teachers suggest that it's unrealistic to expect people to use themselves well in complex activities like singing, piano playing or dancing until they can sit down and stand up without unnecessary tension.

What is the purpose of lying down work?

Alexander himself rarely did lying down work, relegating the task to his assistant teachers. Nevertheless, he obviously deemed it valuable, as it gives the pupil an opportunity to experience a new alignment and integration of mind and body. Compared to sitting, standing, walking and other more complicated activities, lying horizontally with the knees up and the head on a pile of books makes it much easier to harmonize with gravity. A proper lying down lesson still requires the student to inhibit and direct, but the support of the table or floor minimizes the stimulus to misuse. In other words, there is less to inhibit. Thus, the pupil is often better able to assimilate the subtleties of direction communicated by the teacher's hands.

In my own practice I find that many students arrive for their lessons so tired and stressed that they are not able to do the thinking-in-activity that the Alexander work requires. I often find that, after working with my pupils on the table or floor for fifteen minutes or so, their ability to learn and apply the Technique in movement improves dramatically.

Will most of my learning take place during the lesson?

The major learning of the Alexander Technique does not take place during the lesson with the teacher. Rather, *the teacher helps the student develop the tools for learning* by communicating an experience of improved use and an understanding of the role of inhibition and direction in bringing it about.

At the end of a lesson, students usually report feeling lighter, freer and taller. But when the student leaves the teaching room and gets in the car or on a bicycle or bus to go home, the most important learning begins: as he goes back to his normal activities, the stimulus toward habit returns, threatening the integrity of the new, balanced state. The difference is that now, when the student pulls his head back as he pushes down on the bicycle pedal or accelerator or takes that first step onto the bus, he'll be much more likely to notice it. This happens because the lesson raises the awareness of unnecessary tensions and thus makes them susceptible to the power of inhibition. The most important learning of the Technique takes place as the student applies inhibition and direction to the activities of daily life.

Can I keep that lovely Alexander feeling by holding my head in the right position?

One of the paradoxes of learning the Technique is that the surest way to lose the feeling of lightness and ease is to try, directly, to keep it. Moreover, the concept of position, like the concept of posture, is fundamentally static and not very useful to anyone interested in improving their coordination. If you are trying to hold 'the right position' you will stiffen and shorten. If you are trying to 'recreate a feeling' you are living in the past.

The Alexander work takes place *now*, in the ever-changing, present moment. It requires that we focus more on 'letting go' and 'being' than 'holding on' and 'doing'. It invites a never-ending process of applying inhibition and direction to the choices we make regarding the use of ourselves.

No matter how much I work on myself it never feels the same as when a teacher is helping me: why?

Many people feel that they must not be applying the Technique effectively because they cannot create for themselves the same feeling that they get from the hands of a teacher. My advice is: do not even try. Trying to recreate a feeling will not improve your Use. Furthermore, the quality of feeling you get from working with a teacher will tend to be different from that you experience independently. That is a by-product of the impact of a highly trained nervous system on your own.

Different qualities of feeling or sensation can provide useful feedback for your learning process. Notice your changing feelings and their relationship to the choices you make about how you use yourself and avoid being seduced into making a *specific* feeling state your primary focus or sole criterion for progress.

If it is easier for me to relax with my eyes closed, why does the teacher insist that I keep them open?

The Alexander Technique is not relaxation training. When you close your eyes and think about relaxing, your muscle tone becomes less lively, your balance is compromised and your attention is likely to wander.

The Alexander work aims to enliven your muscle tone, sharpen your balance and refine your power of attention. Alert, gently focused eyes promote these conditions.

Is it necessary to understand anatomy to practice the Alexander Technique?

Alexander once met with a group of well-known anatomists who were assembled by some of his supporters to develop an understanding of how and why the Technique worked. When Alexander saw how poorly the anatomists used themselves, however, he walked out of the meeting.

Nevertheless, a practical understanding of living anatomy is a useful complement to your Alexander work. As you gain specific insights into the working of your bones and muscles you can use them more intelligently. You can develop your self-knowledge and improve your Use as you investigate questions such as: Where does my head balance on my neck? What is the role of the sub-occipital muscles? Where is the centre of gravity of my head? of my whole body? Where exactly are my hip joints? Where are my lungs and in what direction does my diaphragm move when I exhale?

I learned recently, for example, that the bones of the sternum are designed as a flexible, seamed structure, not as a rigid palette. As a result, when I think about letting my torso lengthen and widen, my thought now 'contains' the idea that my chest is more flexible than I previously imagined, and a freer, more natural Use tends to emerge.

There is much to be learned from contemplating a skeleton and studying a good anatomy book (I recommend *The Anatomy Colouring Book* by Kapit and Elson, *Albinus on Anatomy* by Hale and Coyle and the 'Body Mapping' chapters in Barbara and Bill Conable's *How to Learn the Alexander Technique* (see Bibliography, pages 166–174). Apply what you learn to improving your Use.

• • •

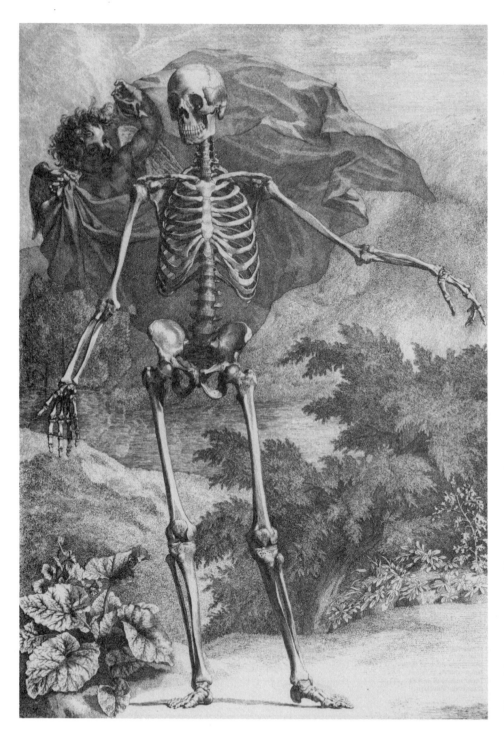

The anatomical drawings of Bernhard Siegfried Albinus (1697–1770) are admired by artists worldwide. Painters and sculptors know that a profound understanding of anatomy deepens artistic perception and expression. An appreciation of practical anatomy can be equally valuable in the arts of movement and self-expression.

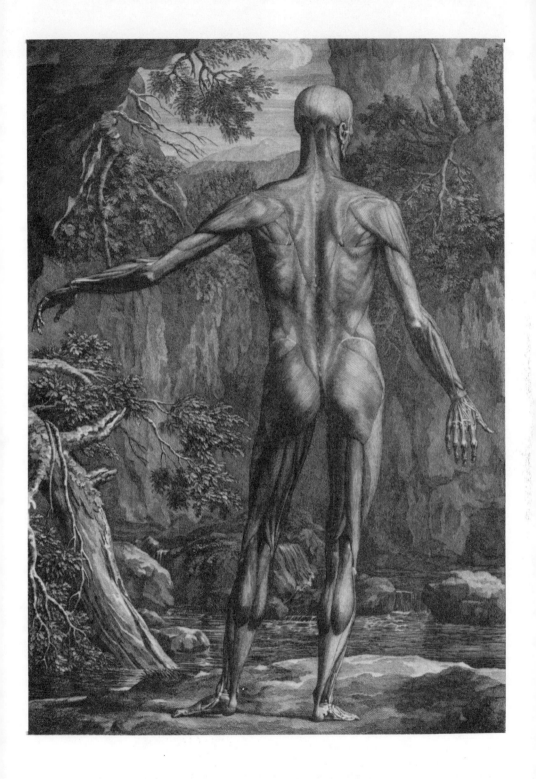

Is exercise incompatible with the Alexander Technique?

Alexander observed that most people perform exercises without considering the question of Use. He was highly critical of the 'no pain, no gain' approach of the 'physical culturists' of his day who promoted distorted, exaggerated muscularity and unnatural methods of breathing. He never opposed exercising, just the unintelligent practice of it.

The understanding of cardiovascular fitness and weight training methods has come a long way since Alexander's time. It should nevertheless be obvious that running or weightlifting without proper attention to poise and balance will do more harm than good.

Regular exercise (preferably activities that you actually *enjoy*) is vital to healthy living. But whatever form or forms you choose, your use of yourself must be taken into account. Apply the Alexander Technique to prevent exercise from harming you while maximizing its benefits and your enjoyment.

Is the AT posture training?

No. The concept of 'posture training' is fundamentally flawed because it suggests a division of mind and body and implies stasis. Moreover, when most people think of 'improving their posture' they stiffen up for a few moments before collapsing again. Our 'postures' are always a reflection of how we use ourselves. The Alexander Technique offers training in the use of the self. Alexander used the word self because it was the best English word to suggest the idea of the whole person. Alexander lessons are not focused on correcting your posture, rather they invite you to apply a new way of thinking that can lead you to the discovery of your *full stature*.

Do you recommend group classes in the Technique?

Group classes provide a valuable adjunct to private lessons. Group work does not, however, replace them. The in-depth, personalized nature of private lessons is essential to the process of incorporating the Alexander work. Nevertheless, group classes offer a number of benefits:

• • •

- For students working on performance problems, a group makes it easy to simulate the reality of stage fright and to receive feedback on the effect of changes in Use on an audience.
- A group setting provides a real opportunity to develop one's power of observation, a skill which was essential to Alexander's discovery of the Technique. Many pupils find that they are better able to recognize and inhibit their own patterns of misuse after seeing them in others.
- A group offers obvious advantages for learning practical anatomy and physiology.
- Group work makes it clear that we are all in the same boat. Many pupils are encouraged and inspired by watching others work on challenges similar to their own.
- The social, collegial atmosphere of a group can make learning more enjoyable and fun.

Effective group teaching requires that the teacher first be skilled in the use of her hands and competent in giving private lessons. A case in point is the work of Marjory Barstow, one of the master teachers of the Alexander Technique, who specializes in group teaching. A graduate of Alexander's first training course, Barstow combines her own brand of midwestern-USA-zen-socratic method with uncanny observational talent and supreme skill in using her hands. Her students receive a profound experience of improved Use while being strongly encouraged to take responsibility for their own learning process.

Do you recommend combining the Alexander Technique with various forms of therapy?

Although the Alexander Technique can be applied effectively to any discipline, there's a major difference between applying and combining and mixing. A number of practitioners have attempted to 'mix' Alexander work with a variety of therapies (from Feldenkrais and Gestalt to cranio-sacral and neo-Reichian therapy), hoping for synergy. The result is usually a hodgepodge that is neither one thing or the other. Trying to be all things to all people is a reliable formula for failure.

Of course, most of us need all the help we can get. There are many valuable therapeutic approaches that serve the quest for wholeness. But I suggest that, with rare exceptions, each discipline is best pursued under independent auspices.

How does the AT differ from Rolfing and other forms of deep tissue bodywork?

When applied by those skilled enough to work painlessly, Rolfing and other forms of deep tissue bodywork can be useful forms of therapy. A Rolfer can be compared to a mechanic who adjusts your car's alignment, cleans out corrosion and repairs dents. An Alexander teacher trains the driver to drive in such a way as to prevent misalignment, corrosion and dents while maximizing the performance of the engine.

What is the difference between the Alexander Technique and the Feldenkrais Method?

The Feldenkrais Method has two aspects: Awareness Through Movement and Functional Integration. The former involves directing the attention in association with a sequence of non-habitual body movements to create an experience of more flexibility and body awareness. The latter involves hands-on work toward a similar end. Both are generally pleasant and result in greater relaxation and flexibility in movement. They are not, however, designed to be applied in everyday activity.

The Alexander work, on the other hand, *is* designed to be applied in everyday activity. As I write these words, for example, I am practising the Alexander Technique, inhibiting my tendency to hunch down over the keyboard, while, in the background of my attention, projecting the directions for positively activating the Primary Control. If I want to apply Feldenkrais I have to stop writing, lie down (a few Feldenkrais procedures can be done in a chair but most begin on the floor) and do the non-habitual exercises.

• • •

Eastern systems of martial arts and meditation all seem to emphasize the primary importance of the belly or pelvis as opposed to the head and neck. Can these different emphases be reconciled?

Through my study of aikido and related disciplines, I've developed an ever-deepening appreciation for the role of the pelvis or 'centre' in generating movement power. This area is the wellspring of life and the centre of our vital energy. To liberate and apply its full power, however, we must *first* free our necks. When the neck is free and the head is going forward and up, the whole torso lengthens and widens, thereby freeing the movement of the pelvis. This freedom allows mind and body to work as a coordinated, harmonious whole. In other words, the pelvis is *central* and the head–neck is *primary*.

How does the Alexander Technique affect the emotions?

The Alexander work can have a wide range of effects on the emotions. Most commonly, people report feeling uplifted, buoyant and more confident as a result of lessons. Improved physical balance and equilibrium usually translates into improved emotional balance and equanimity.

Occasionally, pupils experience profound emotional release during a lesson. Most of the Alexander teachers I know create a safe and supportive environment for learning. Alexander pupils receive a level of non-invasive attention and support which is often unique in their experience. This sense of safety and support can allow pupils to feel secure enough to experience emotions that they may be holding beneath the surface. Moreover, as habitual tensions are released during a lesson, pupils will sometimes experience corresponding emotional release. The Alexander work does not aim directly to facilitate emotional release, but when it does occur the principles of the Technique remain valid and useful.

Whatever the emotion, you are better off experiencing it with a free neck, free breathing and open eyes. Anger becomes clearer and less likely to turn into destructiveness. Sadness is fuller, richer and more cathartic. Joy is unhysterical, more complete and natural.

Some people tend to be 'overly emotional' and 'all over the place' while others armour themselves so thoroughly that they seem to have no emotions at all. Wherever you are on the continuum, your emotional life is always expressed through your body. Recent research suggests that your emotions affect your nerves, muscles and immune system from moment to moment. By refining your kinaesthetic sensitivity, the Alexander work offers you the opportunity to become more aware of the subtleties of your emotional experience. And greater awareness is the first step to greater freedom.

Of course, the Alexander work will not, by itself, resolve all your deepest emotional issues, but it can help you find a healthier, more accurate and intelligent experience and expression of emotion. A rich, fulfilling life requires the ability to feel deeply and honestly while choosing your behaviour freely. The Alexander Technique can help you discover this elusive, dynamic balance.

Can the Alexander Technique help me in my relationships with others?

Interpersonal relationships are tremendously complex. But there are a few simple principles and practices that seem to bring out the best in our communication with others and the Alexander work is relevant to each of them.

- *Listening and understanding are the 'primary control' of successful communication.* If you discipline yourself to inhibit the tendency to talk first, to impose your views, to interrupt and to think of your own reply as someone else speaks, you will be truly able to listen. Listening *first* allows you to express yourself with greater intelligence, and your receptive listening communicates a message of caring and respect that brings out the best in others.

- Many problems in relationships come from our frustration at being unable to change others. 'If only my boss were a better listener.' 'If only my husband were more sensitive.' 'If only my wife understood me better.'

156

The desire to change others stems from a tendency to blame them. Many people, for example, approach relationships with a 'victim' orientation, an orientation that becomes a self-fulfilling prophecy: 'I never get any respect at work', 'Men are jerks', 'My girlfriends always dump me'. Most of us discover, however, that trying to change others directly does not work.

The fundamental message of Alexander's work is that we must take responsibility for ourselves. We may not be able to change others but we can change our manner of responding. And the changes we make in ourselves open a door to bringing out the best in others. Letting your neck be free as your head goes forward and up and your torso lengthens and widens will not magically sort out your relationship problems. But it helps to put the emphasis where it belongs – on changing yourself.

It may be naive to believe that we 'create our own reality' but we certainly affect it dramatically. This is true whether it is a matter of using one's voice well or getting along with others. As my friend and colleague Violet Arnold says: *'We teach others how to treat us'*.

- A significant proportion of our communication is non-verbal. Much of our intuition about people, for example, is the result of reading their body language. Professor Albert Mehrabian and others have demonstrate that if there is any discrepancy between our words and our body language people are much more likely to be influenced by the body language. In other words, your facial expression, gestures and movements frequently communicate more than your words. *The Alexander Technique raises your awareness of the subtleties of body language*, both your own and that of others. It extends your awareness of the 'signals' you send to others and can make you much more sensitive to the 'signals' others are sending to you. This awareness often provides a 'missing link' to effective communication and happier relationships.

•••

How does one reconcile Alexander's emphasis on 'the means-whereby' with the idea of setting and achieving goals in life?

Alexander's warnings about the dangers of 'endgaining' are sometimes misinterpreted to suggest that goals are not important and may actually be counterproductive. This is absurd. Instead, Alexander emphasizes the importance of an intelligent, holistic approach to achieving goals. He challenges us to reassess our goals: are they disconnected products of our conditioning and habit, or reasoned, conscious, integrated choices?

Wise men and women know that happiness is not attained by the direct pursuit of happiness but rather as a by-product of healthy self-expression, appreciation of beauty and service to others. Alexander was a wise man who encouraged balancing goals and processes, ends and means, reason and feeling.

I'm all in favour of personal growth, but in the meantime my neck is stiff and my back hurts. Will the Alexander Technique help?

Back pain and stiff neck are frequently the direct result of misuse. Of course, misuse is not always the primary cause of aches and pains, but it complicates most maladies through what Dewey called 'compensatory maladjustment'. When misuse is the primary cause of a problem, the Alexander Technique will often have a profoundly positive effect. If the issue of Use is secondary, then the Technique will still tend to be helpful, but perhaps in a less dramatic fashion.

If pain relief is your primary motivation for seeking Alexander lessons, consult your physician or primary health care provider; inform your Alexander teacher about your problem (remember, the Technique works indirectly by focusing on improving your Use – do not expect a diagnosis or direct treatment from your Alexander teacher); and read *Back Trouble* by Alexander teacher and physical therapist, Deborah Caplan (see Bibliography, page 167).

Can the Alexander Technique help me sleep better?

Sleep is the domain of what Alexander would have called 'instinctive guidance'. You cannot, of course, inhibit and direct while you are asleep. But you can do so as you prepare for bed and when you arise. Many students find that their sleep improves if they take ten minutes to practice the 'Balanced Resting State Procedure' (see page 161) prior to sleeping and upon arising. Moreover, as you practice the Alexander Technique in your waking hours you may find that the growing sense of well-being that you experience throughout your day translates into more restful sleep.

I also recommend that you invest in the biggest bed that you can afford – to give yourself maximum room to stretch out and roll around in the night. Find the level of mattress firmness, types of pillows and sleep positions that work best for you. Create in your bedroom an environment that is as peaceful and aesthetically pleasing as possible. Listen to soothing music or read your favourite book as you drift off. Pleasant dreams!

Do you have any other thoughts on how I can get more from my Alexander work?

- Seek first to inhibit, then direct.
- Cultivate a questing, experimentally-oriented state of mind.
- Read and contemplate the 'Evolution of a Technique' chapter in Alexander's *The Use of the Self* (see Bibliography, page 166).
- Observe yourself in action, non-judgementally, in a mirror or on video.
- Be fully present, keep your eyes alive and focused.
- Remember that your head and body are three-dimensional.
- Be a student of poise – observe animals, babies, native peoples, great artists and athletes.
- Practice the Balanced Resting State Procedure for ten to twenty minutes every day (see page 161).
- After your first thirty lessons try working with different teachers.
- Combine a deep commitment to learning, growth and change with compassion, forgiveness and acceptance of yourself now.
- Maintain your sense of humour.

• • •

Aren't there exercises or other things that I can do to learn the Alexander Technique without a teacher?

When I first submitted the manuscript of *Body Learning* to my publisher I was urged to include some 'how to do it' exercises. Despite admonitions that the book would sell better, I resisted. In putting together this new edition the publishers once again implored me to include more exercises and things for you to do. They explained that numerous books have appeared offering exercises that readers seem to like. I've read a number of these books and some of them do offer exercises in exploring movement, emotion and energy that are intriguing. Some may even provide a valuable adjunct to your study of the Technique. But they are not and will never be a substitute for working with a teacher. Moreover, readers run the risk of being deluded into thinking that they do not need to continue lessons because they are doing the exercises in the books, and that *what they are doing is what was meant*.

If you are having lessons with a good teacher you do not need a 'how to do it' book and if you are not having lessons, then what you learn from the book may be interesting, perhaps even valuable, but it won't be the Alexander Technique.

Nevertheless, after resisting my publisher's pleas for fifteen years I've decided to reveal the **Ultimate Alexander Exercise**: sit quietly in a chair, preferably in front of a mirror, and reflect on the quality of your life. Consider whether you are really interested in embracing a fundamental process of growth and change. If the answer is yes, then pause, rise to your full stature, walk over to your telephone and call the Society of Teachers of the Alexander Technique and arrange to have lessons.

In the meantime, you might want to try the Balanced Resting State Procedure.

The Balanced
Resting State Procedure

In 1977, when I was in my second year of training as an Alexander teacher, my mother and father visited the training course. Although both my parents supported my choice to train as an Alexander teacher, my father was sceptical about the value of the Technique. As an oral surgeon he was steeped in the Western medical tradition and questioned the validity of the concept of Use.

In addition to spending eight hours a day bending over to operate on people's mouths, it was not unusual for my dad to be called out of bed at 3 a.m. to repair the jaw of someone who'd been shot or hit with an axe. I was not too surprised, therefore, when he said he had been experiencing persistent back pain that was not responding to conventional treatment.

Although sceptical, my dad was willing to try something new. I gave him one Alexander lesson and taught him the Balanced Resting State Procedure. He agreed to practice it twice a day for the next few weeks. He has in fact practised it regularly for the last sixteen years. His back pain (and his scepticism) disappeared within a few days and have not returned. Although the effects of this procedure are not always quite so dramatic, almost everyone finds it helpful and it is most unlikely to cause any harm.

This procedure is known variously as 'constructive resting', 'lying down in semi-supine', just plain 'lying down' or 'the Balanced Resting State procedure'. Practise it two or three times a day for five to fifteen minutes at a time.

All you need to benefit from this procedure is a relatively quiet, warm place, some carpeted floor space, and a few paperback books. To get the most benefit, ask your Alexander teacher to guide you through this process.

- Begin by placing the books on the floor. (Most people require a small pile of books 2–6" (5–15cm) in height. To approximate the right height for you: stand upright with your buttocks and shoulder blades against a wall and measure the distance from the wall to the back of your head, then add ½–1"(1–2½ cm). Stand your body's length away from the books with your feet shoulder-width apart. Let your hands rest gently at your sides. Facing away from the books, look straight ahead with a soft, alert focus. Pause for a few moments.
- Become aware of the contact of your feet on the floor and notice the distance from your feet to the top of your head. Keep your eyes open and alive, and listen to the sounds around you.
- Maintaining this expansive awareness, move lightly and quickly so that you are resting on one knee. Then roll yourself back so that you are supporting yourself with your hands behind you, feet in front and flat on the floor, knees bent. Avoid holding your breath.
- Let your head drop forward a tiny bit to ensure that you are not tightening your neck muscles and pulling your head back. Then gently roll your spine along the floor so that your head rests on the books. The books should be positioned so that they support your head at the place where your neck ends and your head begins. If your head is not well positioned, then pause, reach back with one hand and support your head while using the other hand to place the books in the proper position. Your feet remain flat on the floor, with your knees pointing up to the ceiling and your hands resting on the floor or loosely folded on your chest. Allow the weight of your body to be fully supported by the floor.
- Avoid fidgeting or wriggling around to 'get comfortable'. If you are uncomfortable then start over from the beginning. All you need to reap the benefit of this procedure is to rest in this position. As you rest, gravity will be lengthening your spine while 'undoing' unnecessary twists and tensions. Keep your eyes open to avoid dozing off. You may wish to bring your attention to the flow of your breathing (without trying to change it) and to the gentle pulsation of your whole body. Be

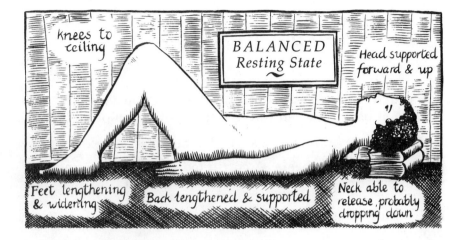

knees to
ceiling

BALANCED
Resting State
~

Head supported
forward & up

Feet lengthening
& widening

Back lengthened & supported

Neck able to
release, probably
dropping down

aware of the ground supporting your back, allowing your shoulders to rest as your back widens. Let your neck be free as your whole body lengthens and expands.

- After you have rested for ten to twenty minutes, get up slowly, being careful to avoid stiffening or shortening your body as you return to a standing position. In order to achieve a smooth transition, decide when you are going to move and then gently roll over on to your front, maintaining your new integration and expansion. Ease your way into a crawling position and then on to one knee. With your head leading the movement upward, stand.
- Pause for a few moments… listen… eyes alive. Again, feel your feet on the floor, and notice the distance between your feet and the top of your head. You may be surprised to discover that the distance has expanded. As you move into the activities of your day, think about 'not doing' anything that interferes with this expansion, ease and overall buoyancy.

For best results, practice the Balanced Resting State when you wake up in the morning, when you come home from work and before retiring at night. The procedure is especially valuable *prior* to giving a presentation or performance, engaging in a competition or meeting to resolve a conflict with a loved one or boss, or before any activity that may be stress-inducing.

Glossary

Constructive conscious control Taking responsibility for the intelligent use of the self through the application of inhibition and direction.

Debauched kinaesthesia A corrupted and therefore untrustworthy sense of position, tension and movement.

Endgaining Grasping for results without thoughtful attention to process.

Functioning The ability to perform according to design.

Inhibition Conscious thinking that prevents interference with the natural alignment and best functioning of our equipment-for-motion.

Leaving yourself alone Allowing yourself to be moved without collapsing or resisting.

Means-whereby, attention to the Focus on the appropriate process to achieve a goal.

Neck to be free, head forward and up, back to lengthen and widen The 'orders' or 'directions' of the Alexander Technique for the proper functioning of the Primary Control. To be projected 'all together, one after the other'. Let's consider them individually:

> **Neck to be free:** releasing *unnecessary* tension in the neck, particularly in the sub-occipital muscles.

> **Head forward and up:** the natural direction of the head; forward means not unnaturally pulled back and up is the opposite of down!

Back to lengthen and widen: the three-dimensional expansion of the torso which follows naturally from a free neck and forward-and-up direction of the head.

Non-doing Avoiding interference with reflex functioning.

Poise Grace under pressure. The right amount of energy in the right place at the right time.

Primary Control The dynamic relationship of the head, neck and torso that organizes our movement and alertness.

Psycho-physical re-education The discipline of unlearning maladaptive habits of use.

Pulled down The state of physical collapse and compromised alertness resulting from interference with the natural functioning of our anti-gravity musculature.

Relax To slacken or loosen.

Self The complex of body, mind and emotion.

Startle pattern The prototypical bio-mechanical response to fear, beginning with contraction of the neck muscles.

Unreliable sensory appreciation Distortion of the senses, especially kinaesthesia, caused by misuse.

Use The power of choice, especially as it applies to our equipment-for-motion.

Bibliography

The Alexander Technique

F.M. Alexander, *The Alexander Technique*, ed. Edward Maisel, Thames & Hudson, London, 1974.
This anthology, which contains Alexander's essential writings and a critical introduction by the editor, is particularly valuable because it also includes the three introductions by John Dewey to Alexander's books.

F.M. Alexander, *Man's Supreme Inheritance*, Dutton, New York, 1910.
Alexander's first book, widely read and acclaimed when it was first published. The major theme is 'the great phase in Man's advancement in which he passes from subconscious to conscious control of his own mind and body'.

F.M. Alexander, *Constructive Conscious Control of the Individual*, Methuen, London, 1923.
Alexander's second book, in which he introduced the concepts of 'endgaining' and 'sensory appreciation'. It also contains a detailed description of procedures used in a typical lesson.

F.M. Alexander, *The Use of the Self*, Dutton, New York, 1932.
A short work centred on a thorough account of the author's discovery of the Technique and introducing the terms 'Use' and 'Primary Control'. Its succinct and direct nature makes this Alexander's best book.

F.M. Alexander, *The Universal Constant in Living*, Dutton, New York, 1941.
Alexander's last book, a hodgepodge of articles and essays devoted to expanding the concept of 'Use'.

166

F.M. Alexander, unpublished autobiographical fragment, London, 1947.

J. Armstrong, 'Effects of the Alexander Principle in Dealing with Stress in Musical Performance', Master's thesis, Tufts University, May 1975.

W. Barlow, *The Alexander Principle*, Victor Gollancz, London, 1973. The chapters on 'Use and Disease' and 'Medical Diagnosis' represent the book's major contribution.

G.C. Bowden, *F. Matthias Alexander and the Creative Advance of the Individual*, L.N. Fowler, London, 1965.
Largely a flight of fancy, this book has two good sections: a brief discussion relating the Alexander experience to Zen in the Art of Archery and the appendix, which contains a journal of lessons with Alexander.

D. Caplan, *Back Trouble: A New Approach to Prevention and Recovery*, Triad Publishing, Gainesville, Florida, 1987.
If you have back trouble this is a book for you.

W. Carrington, 'The F. Matthias Alexander Technique: A Means of Understanding Man', *Systematics*, vol. 1, no. 1, December 1963.
An excellent brief introduction to the Technique.

W. Carrington, 'Balance as a Function of Intelligence', *Systematics*, vol. 7, no. 4, March 1970.
A consideration of the Alexander work in an evolutionary context. This is one of the best articles on the Technique.

W. Carrington and S. Carey, *Explaining the Alexander Technique: The Writings of F.M. Alexander*, The Sheldrake Press, London, 1992.
Sean Carey asks thoughtful, probing questions and Walter Carrington provides informative, charming answers in this marvellous companion to Alexander's books.

B. Conable and W. Conable, *How to Learn the Alexander Technique: A Manual for Students*, Andover Road Press, Columbus, Ohio, 1992.
Despite a tendency toward oversimplification, this manual offers an original and thought-provoking approach to the Alexander work. Especially useful for musicians.

R. Dart, 'The Attainment of Poise', *South African Medical Journal*, vol. 21, February 1947.
Dart wrote this article to explain the Technique to doctors in South Africa; he also wrote papers on the Technique for physical therapists and dentists.

R. Dart, *An Anatomist's Tribute to F. Matthias Alexander*, The Sheldrake Press, London, 1970.
A discussion of the anatomical research which supports Alexander's work.

R.J. Dennis, 'Musical Performance and Respiratory Function in Wind Instrumentalists: Effects of the Alexander Technique on Musculoskeletal Education', Doctoral dissertation, Teachers College, Columbia University, 1987.

G. Doyle, 'The Task of the Violinist: Skill, Stress, and the Alexander Technique', Doctoral dissertation, University of Lancaster, 1984.

F.J.C. Duarte, 'The Principles of the Alexander Technique Applied to Singing: The Significance of the Preparatory Set', Master's thesis, New England Conservatory of Music, 1981.

J.V. Fenton, *Choice of Habit*, Macdonald & Evans, London, 1973.
The only book on the practical applications of the Technique in schools. Fenton presents evidence of the importance of the problem of 'misuse' and offers concrete solutions.

D. Garlick, 'A Physiologist Looks at the Alexander Technique', *AUSTAT Journal*, vol. 1, no. 1, 1986, pp. 4–5.

B. Hamilton, 'The Alexander Technique: A Practical Application to Upper String Playing', Doctoral dissertation, Yale University, 1986.

A. Huxley, *Ends and Means*, Chatto & Windus, London, 1940. In the essay on education, Huxley calls for a 'practical morality working at every level from the bodily to the intellectual' and suggests the Alexander Technique as a means of realizing this goal. The chapter on ethics is also interesting.

A. Huxley, 'End-gaining and Means Whereby', *The Saturday Review of Literature*, October 1941.

A. Huxley, *Letters of Aldous Huxley*, ed. Grover Smith, Chatto & Windus, London, 1969.
References to Alexander are scattered throughout.

F.P. Jones, *Body Awareness in Action, A Study of the Alexander Technique*, Schocken Books, New York, 1976.
Jones emphasizes the educational and moral implications of the Alexander Technique and presents the results of his scientific research, carried out at the Tufts Center for Experimental Psychology, which support Alexander's findings.

F.P. Jones, *Select Papers of Frank Pierce Jones*, ed. Richard Brown, Tufts University, Massachussetts, 1976.

B.G. Levy, 'Somatic Education as an Approach to the Conceptualization and Treatment of Anxiety', Doctoral dissertation, University of California at Berkeley, 1986.

P.P. Lewis, 'The Alexander Technique – Its Relevance for Singers and Teachers', Doctoral dissertation, Carnegie-Mellon University, 1980.

A. Matthews, 'Implications for Education in the Work of F.M. Alexander: An Exploratory Project in a Public School Classroom', Master's thesis, Bank Street College of Education, 1984.

E.D. McCormack, 'Frederick Matthias Alexander and John Dewey: A Neglected Influence', Doctoral dissertation, University of Toronto, 1956.
The author shows that Dewey's support for Alexander reflected 'his deep conviction that Alexander was correct' and that the Technique contained 'the promise and potentiality of the direction that is needed in all education'.

P. Sanfillipo, 'A Reader's Guide to the Alexander Technique: A Selected Annotated Bibliography', Master's thesis, University of Wisconsin at Madison, 1982.

C. Stevens, *Alexander Technique*, Optima, London, 1987.
A practical, accessible introductory manual with delightful cartoon illustrations by Shaun Williams.

I. Tasker, 'An Unrecognised Need in Education', *South African Journal of Science*, vol. 39, 1947.
A good introduction to the Technique which stresses the importance of an approach to education based on mind–body unity and 'non-endgaining'.

N. Tinbergen, 'Ethology and Stress Disease', *Science*, vol. 185, no. 4145, 1974.
This speech, made when Tinbergen accepted his Nobel Prize, describes the benefits he and his family received from the Technique. Tinbergen also praises Alexander's use of scientific method and argues that this approach should be a model for contemporary ethologists and doctors.

L. Westfeldt, *F. Matthias Alexander: The Man and his Work*, Associated Booksellers, Connecticut, 1964.
Lulie Westfeldt was one of the first people trained to teach the Technique. Although this book is unique and fascinating, it is rather more an autobiography than a biography.

Related topics

T. Buzan, *Use Your Head*, BBC Publications, London, 1976.
A useful book synthesizing a variety of approaches to learning, memory training, speed reading and note taking. It contains excellent practical exercises.

T. Buzan, *The Mind Map Book: Radiant Thinking*, BBC Books, London, 1993.
Mind mapping is the ultimate tool for developing a perception and understanding of 'wholes' and this is the ultimate book on the subject.

G.E. Coghill, *Anatomy and the Problem of Behaviour*, Cambridge University Press, 1949.
Coghill's major work.

J. Dewey, *Human Nature and Conduct*, Modern Library, New York, 1930.
The chapters on habit show a strong Alexandrian influence.

J. Dewey, *John Dewey on Education*, ed. Reginald Archambault, Modern Library, New York, 1964.
A selection of Dewey's writings on education including a statement of his 'Pedagogic Creed'.

J. Dewey, *Experience and Education*, Collier Books, New York, 1972.
A concise statement of Dewey's theory of experience and its relevance to his philosophy of education.

J. Fagan and I.L. Shepherd (eds), *Gestalt Therapy Now,* Penguin Books, Harmondsworth, 1970.
A collection of articles and case histories by 21 Gestalt therapists.

M. Feldenkrais, *Body and Mature Behaviour*, International Universities Press, New York, 1973.
A study of the physiological mechanisms behind the human 'anti-

gravity system' and their relation to functioning. Feldenkrais's work was clearly influenced by his exposure to the Alexander Technique.

D. Garlick (ed.), 'Personal Health and Well Being', Committee in Postgraduate Medical Education, University of New South Wales, 1977.

D. Garlick (ed.), 'Proprioception, Posture and Emotion', Committee in Postgraduate Medical Education, University of New South Wales, 1982.
Dr Garlick appears to be picking up where Frank Pierce Jones left off.

M. Gelb, *Present Yourself: The Simple Way to Give Powerful and Effective Presentations*, Aurum Press, London, 1988.
Applications of mind mapping and Alexander work to this important skill.

M. Gelb and T. Buzan, *Lessons from the Art of Juggling: How to Achieve your Full Potential in Business, Learning and Life*, Harmony Books, New York, 1994.
A guide to learning how to learn based on Alexanderian thought and practice.

M. Gelb, *Mind Mapping: How to Liberate Your Natural Genius*, (audio cassette programme). Available from Nightingale-Conant Co., 7300 North Leigh Avenue, Niles, Illinois 60714.
This bestselling audio programme will train you to be a mind mapper and systems thinker.

R.B. Hale and T. Coyle, *Albinus on Anatomy*, Dover, New York, 1988.
The human form described through a magical synthesis of science and art.

E. Herrigel, *Zen in the Art of Archery*, with an introduction by D.T. Suzuki, Vintage Books, New York, 1971.

This wonderful book describes the experiences of a German professor who spent seven years studying the Zen mysteries. Herrigel puts forward the idea of 'non-doing', which is strikingly similar to Alexander's concept of 'inhibition'.

J. Holt, *Freedom and Beyond*, Penguin Books, Harmondsworth, 1972.
Holt argues that genuine educational freedom is an inner state rather than merely an external relaxation of constraints and goes on to show how the schooling process stifles this inner freedom.

J. Holt, *How Children Fail*, Penguin Books, Harmondsworth, 1974.
An extraordinary collection of observations and insights on contemporary schooling. The author demonstrates that fear and 'endgaining' pervade the educational system.

J. Holt, *How Children Learn*, Penguin Books, Harmondsworth, 1975.
Particularly valuable for the insights into the way children think. Holt describes his own experiences of learning to think 'like a child' and asks educators and psychologists to 'look at children, patiently, repeatedly, respectfully, and to hold off making theories and judgements about them until they have in their minds what most of them do not now have – a reasonably accurate model of what children are like.'

J. Holt, *Instead Of Education*, Penguin Books, Harmondsworth, 1976.
A powerful book that questions the assumptions upon which our educational system is based.

W. Kapit and L. Elson, *The Anatomy Colouring Book*, HarperCollins, New York, 1977.
A marvellous 'whole-brain' approach to learning anatomy.

B. Libet, 'Time of Conscious Intention to Act in Relation to Onset of Cerebral Activity (Readiness-Potential)', *Brain*, no. 106, 1983, from the Neurological Institute, Department of Neuroscience,

Mount Zion Hospital and Medical Center, the Department of Physiology, School of Medicine, and the Department of Statistics, University of California at Berkeley.
Libet's work has tremendous implications for the understanding of the mechanism of inhibition and direction.

R.E. Ornstein, *The Evolution of Consciousness: The Origins of the Way We Think*, Touchstone Books, New York, 1991.
Brain researcher Ornstein emphasizes that, as a species, our days of 'unconscious adaption' are over. He makes a fascinating and compelling case for the necessity of 'constructive conscious control'.

O.W. Sacks, *The Man Who Mistook His Wife for a Hat*, Duckworth, London, 1985.
Chapter three, 'The Disembodied Lady', presents a chilling look at life without proprioception.

M. Saotome, *Aikido and the Harmony of Nature*, Shambhala, Boston, 1993.
If the Alexander Technique were a martial art it would be aikido. This book offers a thorough expression of aikido philosophy.

P. Senge, *The Fifth Discipline: The Art and Practice of the Learning Organization*, Currency Books, New York, 1990.
Alexander said that individuals always function as a whole and can only be changed as such; Senge shows that the same is true for organizations.

M. Sharaf, *Fury on Earth: A Biography of Wilhelm Reich*, St Martin's Press/Marek, New York, 1983.
A compelling biography of one of the century's most underrated geniuses. Reich developed the concept of 'character armour', and pioneered the body–mind approach to psychotherapy.

Notes

1. Frank Jones, 'Method for Changing Stereotyped Response Patterns by the Inhibition of Certain Postural Sets', *Psychological Review*, 3 (May 1965).
2. Frank Jones, *Body Awareness in Action: a Study of the Alexander Technique* (Schocken Books, New York, 1976), p. 2.
3. Leo Stein in Frank Jones, *Body Awareness in Action*, p. 48.
4. John Dewey in F.M. Alexander, *Constructive Conscious Control of the Individual* (Integral Press, London, 1955), pp. xxvii–xxviii.
5. John Dewey in F.M. Alexander, *The Use of the Self* (Integral Press, London, 1945), p. xviii.
6. John Dewey in F.M. Alexander, *Constructive Conscious Control of the Individual*, p. xxvii.
7. Nikolaas Tinbergen, 'Ethology and Stress Diseases', *Science*, 185:4145 (1974), p. 28.
8. F.M. Alexander, *The Use of the Self*, p. 10.
9. *Ibid*, p. 10.
10. *Ibid*, p. 14.
11. Walter Carrington, 'The F. Matthias Alexander Technique: a Means for Understanding Man', *Systematics*, 1 (December 1963), p. 235.
12. F.M. Alexander, *The Universal Constant in Living* (E. P. Dutton, New York, 1941), p. 8.
13. Herbert Spencer in F.M. Alexander, *Man's Supreme Inheritance* (Chaterson, London, 1946), p. 194.
14. Wilfred Barlow, *The Alexander Principle* (Arrow, London, 1975), p. 103.
15. Frank Jones, *Body Awareness in Action*, p. 14.
16. *Ibid*, p. 97.
17. John Dewey, *Human Nature and Conduct* (Modern Library, New York, 1930), p. 31.
18. John Dewey, 'Preoccupation with the Disconnected', *Alexander Journal*, 3 (spring 1964), p. 11.

19. Sir Charles Sherrington, *The Endeavour of Jean Fernel* (Cambridge University Press, 1946), p. 89.

20. Raymond Dart, 'The Attainment of Poise', *South African Medical Journal*, 21 (February 1947), pp. 74–91.

21. Walter Carrington, 'Balance as a Function of Intelligence', *Systematics*, 7 (March 1970), p. 8.

22. Sir Charles Sherrington, *The Endeavour of Jean Fernel*, p. 89.

23. John Dewey in F.M. Alexander, *The Use of the Self*, p. xxi.

24. Rudolf Magnus in Walter Carrington, 'The F. Matthias Alexander Technique: A Means for Understanding Man', p. 243.

25. Frank Jones, 'The Organisation of Awareness', paper read at a conference on *Coordination in Music* at Michigan State University (May 1967), p. 9.

26. Nikolaas Tinbergen, 'Ethology and Stress Diseases', p. 28.

27. John Dewey in F.M. Alexander, *Constructive Conscious Control of the Individual*, p. xxi.

28. Sir Charles Sherrington, *The Integrative Action of the Nervous System* (Cambridge University Press, 1952), p. 196.

29. Sir Charles Sherrington in Frank Jones, 'A Mechanism for Change', *Collected Papers of Frank Jones* (Tufts University, Boston, 1975), p. 185.

30. Frank Jones, 'Changing Stereotyped Response Patterns', *Collected Papers*, p. 27.

31. F.M. Alexander, *Man's Supreme Inheritance*, p. 21.

32. F.M. Alexander, 'Teaching Aphorisms', *Alexander Journal*, 7 (spring 1972), p. 43.

33. D'Arcy Thompson in Frank Jones, *Body Awareness in Action*, p. 139.

34. John Basmajian, 'Conscious Control of Single Nerve Cells', *New Scientist*, 369 (December 1963), p. 663.

35. F.M. Alexander in Frank Jones, *Body Awareness in Action*, p. 165.

36. John Dewey, *Human Nature and Conduct*, pp. 28–30.

37. *Ibid*, pp. 30–37.

38. Aldous Huxley, 'Endgaining and Means Whereby', *Alexander Journal*, 4 (spring 1965), p. 19.

39. Eugen Herrigel, *Zen in the Art of Archery* (Vintage Books, New York, 1971), p. 71.

40. D.T. Suzuki in Eugen Herrigel, *Zen in the Art of Archery*, p. 12.

41. John Holt, *How Children Fail* (Penguin, Harmondsworth, 1974), p. 165.

42. *Ibid*

43. F.M. Alexander, 'Teaching Aphorisms', *Alexander Journal*, 7 (spring 1972), p. 43.

44. Aldous Huxley, 'Endgaining and Means Whereby', *Alexander Journal*, 4 (spring 1965), p. 23.

45. John Dewey in Wilfred Barlow, 'Editorial', *Alexander Journal*, 6 (summer 1968), p. 1.

46. Irene Tasker, 'An Unrecognised Need in Education', *Alexander Journal*, 6 (summer 1968), p. 9.

47. Joyce Warrack, 'Irene Tasker on Education Without Endgaining', *Alexander Journal*, 2 (summer 1963), p. 21.

48. Joyce Roberts, 'Tribute to Miss Tasker', *Alexander Journal*, 6 (summer 1968), p. 4.

49. Jack Fenton, *Choice of Habit* (Macdonald & Evans, London, 1973), pp. 11–30.

50. John Dewey in F.M. Alexander, *Constructive Conscious Control of the Individual*, p. xxviii.

Useful Addresses

United Kingdom
The Society of Teachers of the Alexander Technique (STAT), 20 London House, 266 Fulham Road, London SW10 9EL; tel. (071) 351 0828.

USA
North American Society of Teachers of the Alexander Technique (NASTAT), PO Box 112484, Tacoma, WA 98411-2484; tel. (206) 627 3766.

Australia
Australian Society of Teachers of the Alexander Technique (AUSTAT), PO Box 716, Darlinghurst, NSW 2010; tel. (008) 339 571.

Canada
Canadian Society of Teachers of the Alexander Technique, Box 47025, Apt. 12, 555 West 12th Avenue, Vancouver, B.C. V5Z 3X0; tel: (604) 689 9102.

South Africa
South African Society of Teachers of the Alexander Technique (SASTAT), 35 Thornhill Road, Rondebosch 7700; tel. (021) 686 8454.

I particularly recommend the Alexander Technique workshops sponsored by Michael Frederick, PO Box 408, Ojai, California 93024; tel. (805) 646 8902.

Picture acknowledgements

20 The Australian Information Service, London
28 *top:* Brian Moody *bottom:* © Sally and Richard Greenhill
36 *top:* Mike King *bottom:* © Sally and Richard Greenhill
38 By permission of Jules Feiffer and the British Library
40 Donald Greenwood
43 © Anthea Sieveking/Vision International
45 Donald Greenwood
48 © Agence Nature/NHPA
49 © Kennan Ward
55 Mike King
62 Sarah Errington/Hutchison Library
65 *top:* Greg Evans International *bottom:* Camera Press/William MacQuitty
72 Mark Boulton/Barnaby's Picture Library
73 Pierre Berger/Barnaby's Picture Library
76 Sporting Pictures (UK) Ltd
81 Sporting Pictures (UK) Ltd
98 Sporting Pictures (UK) Ltd
163 Fiona White

Index